Calories & Real Foods Diet

K.J.R. Alexander

CONTENTS

This book is a revised condensed version of Love Your Diet's *Light Fantastic*. See this edition in print for explanatory and informational charts and tables comparing nutritional content in foods.

For protein amounts in foods, see the printed edition of *Calorie Counter* in the Love Your Diet Series.

1 LOVE YOUR DIET

Other Diets – The Fat Comes Back!

In your past experience with the fat struggle, you said to yourself that you needed to lose some weight. Just the thought made you hungry. At first, you may have thought that you just needed healthier food. Then there were all those snapshot diet tips in the media: don't eat high-fructose corn syrup, don't eat gluten, shop the perimeter of the store, cut out that morning sweet coffee confection, eat fruits and vegetables. You may have tried out all these ideas that just didn't do anything. Just like sometimes eating an apple or munching some celery didn't help. The stubborn fat wouldn't budge.

The reason for the lack of punch in such strategies were that these weight loss ideas were only little pieces of the puzzle, a small part of the bigger picture. The people giving the advice were already slender and getting paid for the interesting tips. You learned that the ideas may be nice to try out, but something was missing.

You decided more drastic measures were needed. You looked for a weight loss plan that promised, and delivered, plenty of punishment to torture the hated fat away. With heroic efforts, you maintained the motivation, endured all the hardship, and lost some weight. It was not easy. You were rightly proud of yourself. Then what happened? The fat came back! A lot faster than it came off. You were left with having to do it all over again.

The drama is played out with all kinds of weight loss methods as we try to beat our bodies into submission. Consider more of the common dieting dilemmas. You have probably already tried some of these methods without lasting success.

Just stop eating. This is the most typical short-lived dieting strategy, often a favorite with guys. After all, it is so logical. The problem is that the body immediately shuts down metabolism and goes on "save" when food is

1

suddenly reduced. Survival mode kicks in. After eating hardly anything and going hungry for several days, no weight is lost.

Joining a reducing club that provides low-calorie food at big prices is predictably bad. Not only are you a prisoner without choice, the food is tiny and you are hungry! When you are free to make choices again, you go directly to the fattening foods with new purpose.

Some support groups also have major disadvantages. While sharing your problem with others who also want to change, the pitfall is that it may fix your torture in concrete. The mindset is fixed with only two options: starve or store fat forever. How easy this is to give up in defeated surrender.

Drinking high nutrient diet drinks in place of meals offers convenience and fixed calories, while taking away the choice of foods. The problem is that the body needs to digest real food and you are quickly and constantly hungry. However, these nutritious drinks are good for additional protein and nutritional support while dieting. This means they can work in support of real food.

Diet pills, synthetic metabolic enhancers, and appetite suppressors are not considered safe or healthy choices and must not be used. These substances have been known to cause harm to the liver, heart, lungs, and kidneys. There are no magic pill replacements for the food the body naturally needs.

Heavy exercise. The more the exercise, the more food is metabolized. Olympic and other sports competitors must eat a lot of food to replace the calories they need for high energy activity. With heavy exercise, the body tunes up for survival as though preparing for battling, running, hunting, collecting. For those in shape, it feels good and powerful but requires more and more time and maintenance and more and more food. Looking at buffed-up enthusiasts as examples, you tell yourself you just need more exercise to lose weight.

But think about this for the average person. Playing golf or ballroom dancing uses only about 300 calories per hour. The strenuous activity of mowing the lawn with a hand mower uses about 460 calories per hour. Walking at 2.5 miles per hour utilizes only some 215 calories per hour. In addition, exercise may make you think you can safely eat more because you are exercising. Yet burning off those big pieces of cake you ate at 300-500 calories a slice or that fast food burger meal at 1,000 calories can require anywhere from 2 to 5 hours of exercise. This is just not practical and a no-win situation for most. There is also a risk to health in suddenly exercising an overweight body. This includes damage to joints, cartilage, and muscles as well as heart and vascular stress. You've probably seen your overweight friends on crutches or with bandaged joints from suddenly working out in a short-lived burst of enthusiasm.

This is the reason why gentle to moderate exercise is best at first for serious dieters who are out of shape. Exercise is great for overall health, and yes, modern life is too sedentary and increases weight. Exercise works in support of weight loss. It improves health and attitude while using up some calories. But the point is that more of a game plan than exercise alone is needed for burning off the fat.

Fad diets and strenuous workouts may offer quick weight loss at considerable expense and devotion, but what about the real results? Do you really want to torture yourself and lose weight temporarily, then keep repeating the process? Why does fat keep fighting back? There is a problem here but what is it? Is the dieter really at fault? Or is something wrong with the method? Why don't diets work? The answers are crystal clear once you see the reasons. These are explained more in the following chapters.

Stress and Bad Food

First of all, the biggest problem with diets of all kinds is that they require suffering with hunger or abnormal cravings. This means the diet will fail in the long term because of the feelings of assault to the body. The body has biology with an agenda to battle for survival.

Our modern lives are full of stresses to the body. Food can be a big substitute for love, affection, and socialization. These are emotional stresses. Worrying about money and paying bills can be mental stress. The physical body feels stress with the fatigue from not getting enough sleep. The body feels these inharmonious states as threats not only to security, but as threats to survival. This is why stress diets only add to the problem. The body doesn't distinguish and categorize stress as emotional, mental, or physical. It just wants to prepare for *physical* survival against starvation. And that means eating!

The biological demands for life and growth are centered in constant needs for food and nourishment. Each day, the body needs food and drink for life. But there's a problem with the kind of food available. With the rapid advance of science and industry, food and its production have been industrialized and technologized. New chemicals, food additives, food processing and packaging create new biological demands for the body's adjustment and adaptation.

Highly-refined industrial foods create a body out of balance with its natural needs creating the feelings to satisfy the body by eating more. Yet the food itself is out of whack, out of synchronization, with what the body knows. Now there's a double whammy: the increased stress of modern life and the increased stress of....bad food. Food the body doesn't know how to deal with. That the body does not readily digest industrialized foods is so obvious we may wonder why we don't acknowledge it more in our eating choices. We learn that natural foods are more healthy. But we don't eat as though we believe industrialized, highly-processed foods are addictive and fattening. We even kid ourselves in the confusion of what is really natural.

We expect more from our biology than it is equipped to handle. A good diet needs to decrease stress and bad food, not add more of it.

This diet is none of the things just discussed. It is not about torture, hunger, cravings, packaged food deliveries, and go-til-you-drop exercise, all without delicious carbohydrate foods that are so satisfying.

Love Your Diet

Ask yourself what you need in a diet. In your wildest dreams, you want to eat whatever you want, whenever you want without packing on the fat. But does this include endless chips and candy bars? Does this kind of food really *feel* good? You *can* have the diet of your wildest dreams - a healthy diet that is deeply *satisfying*, tastes wonderful, dissolves fat, then keeps it off. A list of what a diet should help you do would look like this:

Eat delicious satisfying foods

Melt away excess fat without hunger

Control weight after dieting

Stop food addictions

Choose foods that are not fattening

Heal metabolism and make it free

Eat a healthy balanced diet

Diet without spending a fortune

Enjoy food all over again

Eat gourmet on a budget

Replace bad foods with good foods

Eat breads and pastas

Eat safe sweets and safe sugars

Know how to eat fast food and junk food without weight gain

Know how to prepare menu items

Understand why some foods are good and nutritious and others are fat-producers

Eat convenient, safe, on-the-go foods

Eat a huge variety of foods that do not cause weight gain

Not only are these factors desirable, they are necessary for success. This diet answers the call with why and how and more.

As you experience this diet's power and goodwill, you will say to yourself that this is a wonderful diet. You will actually "love your diet" and gladly stay with the plan. And as you love your diet, you will love yourself.

In the future, as you continue the way of eating on your own, without weight gain, without dieting, you'll see that this diet is in-between-and-above, in a space of its own

But getting there requires strategy and defense and informed food choices. With planning, you can have whatever you want, whenever you want, with some guidelines.

The next chapter, *Show Me the Way*, will outline a plan that combines the best dieting strategies.

2 SHOW ME THE WAY

How can all the ideas discussed so far be formed into a diet, an actual eating plan, where you get more of everything: more nutrition, more food, more calories, more natural carbs, more needed protein, more food choices. The diet will be set up in parts that come together.

Not only is this plan comfortable and enjoyable, it will show you how you can eat a banquet of foods and still lose excess fat. Most importantly, you will be able to maintain that weight loss afterwards without effort and without dieting. The weight you lose will be fat and not the water weight that comes right back on other diets. This is healthy weight loss with balanced nutrition. You will steadily lose from at least two to five pounds a week or more of excess unhealthy fat that does not come back. And since it not like dieting, you can easily maintain your eating, including all your favorite foods. This is a diet that shows you how to eat, not how to do without. It is a diet of freedom from dieting. You will be amazed at all the food that is not fattening.

And yes, you do count calories. But in a new way. *And only during weight loss and not after.* The calorie count is not set up on tortuous minimums but on revolutionary hunger versus fat-loss maximums. You will need to weigh yourself *every day* too. These are necessary figures for tracking your eating. Serious weight loss needs calorie-counting and monitoring with the math and science. Otherwise you kid yourself with all kinds of random reasons like "I got more exercise today so I can eat more cake," or "I'm eating healthy food so it doesn't matter if I eat more junk food." By weighing yourself first thing in the morning, you can see for yourself the effects of your choices. You also learn a lot about yourself and about foods. This is all explained more in Chapter 8, *Maximum Calories: The Goldilocks Paradigm*. A calorie counter is available in a separate book, *Counting Calories*. The printed version is easiest to use and includes protein amounts in foods.

This is a diet that lays a foundation of knowledge and understanding enabling planning and strategy more than it is about set menus. After all, if you only followed menus, you would need 365 x 3 of them for 365 days a year. This is not reasonable and you would soon lose interest. It's also way too restrictive in what you can eat. In addition, by relying only on menus, you open yourself up to "whatever" on your "days off" and after the menus are over. With understanding, you are free to make your own menus and your own wise choices. However, starter menu formats are provided in a later chapter. They are designed for you to continue on your own. After you lose the desired weight by making your own decisions with understanding, you will also know how to maintain that weight loss. Understanding the key concepts is crucial to understanding the causes and cures for your weight gain. With that understanding, you can make your own exceptions and know what you can get away with when it comes to the tempting choices in our food environment.

The diet is simple. You need only to follow it. It is put together with a combination of factors that work together in taking off fat and controlling weight comfortably. It changes the approach to dieting and eating with new ideas that work together beautifully. But first, you must look at the whole picture to see how it all fits together. To do that, we're going to look at a formula in letters and then discuss each part of the formula in later chapters to build the strategy, the plan of action.. The first week of menus is also provided. Remember that action follows thought, so you must have the thoughts first.

Here is the strategic plan:

$$SSSA + X(NC + HP + NH + MC) = \text{Fat Loss}$$

The X factor goes with everything inside the parentheses. In other words, the X factor applies to all the others.

Here are what the letters stand for:

SSSA – Stop Starch and Sugar Addiction
X – Secret X Factor
NC – Natural Carbs
HP – High Protein
NH – No Hunger
MC – Maximum Calories

Each of these will be explained in later chapters. For now, we are establishing the overall strategy and defining some of the terms.

What are carbohydrates?

Starch and sugar. Carbohydrates. These can be especially confusing in today's eating. So first, if only as a refresher, we need to sort out the categories of food into carbohydrates, proteins, and fats.

Food Categories		
Carbohydrates	**Proteins**	**Fats**
Grains & grain products Fruits Vegetables *Everything not a protein or a fat.*	Meats Dairy Products Soy Products	Vegetable oil Meat fat Manufactured margarine and shortening

Food is categorized by how it is digested or metabolized in the body in complex chemical processes. Fats are changed into fatty acids, some fat soluble and some water soluble. Proteins are changed into peptides and then to amino acids. Some of these are essential amino acids needed daily in the diet and not manufactured in the body. Carbohydrates are starches that are changed into different types of sugars, such as glucose, galactose, and fructose. Of course, this is an oversimplification, but the point here is that there are different types of sugars in digestion. This understanding will be applied in the diet. Read about sugar digestion online for curiosity's sake, but good luck in understanding all the chemistry. Nutrition and digestive processes are very complex scientific areas that seem to be of little help to the dieter and the average person. However, the main ideas can be condensed and put to work in understanding your own food metabolism. In the next chapter, the beginning of the diet, *SSSA* is explained.

3 SSSA – STOP STARCH AND SUGAR ADDICTION
SSSA + X(NC + HP + NH + MC) = Fat Loss

Stop starch and sugar addiction and stop packing on the pounds. Free yourself. Get out of jail. This is a complicated addiction to manufactured, industrially-created, processed foods, as this diet will prove. The addiction is *not* caused by *natural* starch and sugar, but more on that later. For now, you must understand that certain foods are causing you to eat more and more without satisfaction. Here are some of the symptoms. Note that the first symptom is the most important one.

1. You are overweight and gaining.
2. Eating only creates the need to eat more. Your body can't seem to get enough food. Your mind is saying you are eating too much, but your body wants to eat more.
3. You do not want to eat many fruits and vegetables.
4. You crave fast food and fattening food like hamburgers, french fries, and milkshakes to the exclusion of other foods.
5. You crave convenience food that has been manufactured and processed like chips, cookies, and shelf cakes.
6. You are tired and fatigued all the time.
7. You are exceptionally sleepy after eating.
8. You are depressed.
9. You are stressed.
10. You seek comfort in sweets and more sweets, starch and more starch.

Addiction

Much of the food we eat today is ersatz food, substitute or artificial food. Yet some would still argue that food is food, regardless of its metamorphosis into different forms, that a lot of junky food has vitamins added, and that the biggest problem is that people simply over-indulge.

When it comes to our modern food, most of us figure if it doesn't immediately kill us, it's okay by us. We have a lot more important things to do and to worry about. All of us sometimes, and some of us all the time, take pride in the valor of being impervious to nutritional concerns, charging with gusto into the lusty forays of junky food gastronomy and convenience foods. Yet, consider the effects, the addictive effects, the fat effects.

The experience with refined, manufactured, processed carbohydrates and sugar products is that the more one eats them the more one wants, to the exclusion of healthier foods. Observe anyone, including yourself, who is serious about pursuing obesity, as to how important constant bags of cookies and potato, corn, or cheese chips are. These are fill-ins allowing constant eating between convenience food meals. Add the trips to the fast food restaurants, donut shops, and hamburger stands. It is like an addiction. It *is* an addiction.

Modern food is created by manufacturing and offers long shelf life. The preparation, the cutting, seasoning, mixing, and in some, the cooking, has already been done for the convenience of the customer, who, at most, has only to heat and eat, after conquering the packaging. This industrial food is designed by vast corporate networks to produce profit. With many of these foods, the consumer is enticed by marketing, convenience, and at most, cheap thrills in the taste buds.

The cheap thrills are salt, sugar, hydrogenated fats, and artificial flavors. The flavors are artificial because they are not natural. They are not of the earth but of the chemist's kitchen. The flour ingredients in many of these foods are unnatural too, stripped of nutrients in refining processes, reduced to paste, and used as fillers to resemble food.

The sticky, addictive substances, flour paste, excessive salt, sugar, chemical preservatives and flavorings, and hydrogenated fats, are also the ingredients in many fast foods, which have the same ingredients that are in the supermarket products because they are the cheapest, most profitable, and are purchased from the same manufacturers.

Sticky Gummy Calories

Take a look at someone walking by with a waddle. What are they eating? They are eating sticky gummy calories. You can "see" the cookies, chips, and crackers. If you are overweight, most likely it is because you too are eating sticky gummy calories. This is food that sticks to you like glue. To your thighs. To your hips. To your stomach. Sticky gummy calories are the starchy carbohydrates and refined sugar in manufactured foods. They are high in oil and salt content and high in strange additive mixtures that do not begin to resemble the original foods. They are made from flour, water, and sugar to form sticky paste. Colors and flavorings are added. These foods are high in calories in relation to the substance and nutrition received from them. They are "empty calories" lacking adequate nutrition and therefore metabolic material.

A good example of nutrients lost in manufacturing is wheat fat or wheat germ oil found in the wheat kernel, the richest known source of vitamin E, a fat soluble antioxidant vitamin, promoting heart and circulatory health, voluntary nerve function, and cell metabolism. The wheat germ and its vitamin E, as well as the nutritious bran exterior of the wheat grain are removed during refining along with B vitamins, protein, and minerals. Only some nutrients are retained or added back in by manufacturers to make enriched flour.

Whole grain nutrients are stripped from grain products during refining to not only extend shelf life but to produce lighter-tasting flour products. Artificial flavors can then more easily be added and more varieties of products fashioned, from breads, cakes, pastries, and cereals to starchy fillers in soups, canned foods, snacks, and frozen dinners. Highly concentrated in empty calories, processed grain products, combined with added starches such as corn starch, along with shortening, leavenings of chemical air, excessive salt, and sugar, are especially devastating to those prone to overweight.

Refined sugar also contains highly concentrated empty calories, while natural sugars such as those in fruits are not concentrated. Refined concentrated sugar has been compared to refined concentrated heroin from the opium poppy, with its own characteristics of addiction. Refined sugar creates a punch, a *sugar high*, or elevated mood and activity level as the body begins to digest it. As the body produces more insulin to utilize the concentrated sugar, a *sugar low* results, with feelings of fatigue and weariness. The result is the alternate high and low characteristic of addictive substances.

The experience with such over-refined carbohydrates and white refined sugar is that the more one eats them, the more one wants. As more is eaten, the body feels increasingly sluggish and sleepy. Hunger is continuous, with vague longings for more starch and sugar products. The dissatisfaction is felt as a need to eat still more, even though the stomach is more than full. The body goes to fat mode.

The distortion of natural nutrition in manufactured food therefore creates instability and hunger as the body misses some of the nutrients. Eating these refined carbohydrates and refined sugars creates addiction. The body *cannot get enough*...of something...needed for metabolism. The chemicals used in foods, as well those left behind as manufacturing residues, are throwing the body out of adjustment. So it is not simply missing nutrients, but the added strange ingredients that make the body feel as though it needs additional metabolic material to deal with the alien substances for which there seems to be no coding.

Consequently, the body, unfamiliar with the new foods, the chemicals and additives, is unable to discard or burn certain substances as fuel, at least not immediately; it simply packs them away like you do all your junk, planning to deal with the problem later. The accumulated junk is fat on the middle, the hips, and then everyplace else on the body. Some of it is water in tissues. And the body (and you) is not going to "deal with it" until there's some kind of break allowing such. When you stop eating excessive sticky gummy calories, the body has more time to deal with the ones it already has in fat.

Stop Starch and Sugar Addiction

The first task of the diet is to *Stop Starch and Sugar Addiction*. This means *refined, manufactured* starch and sugar in highly-processed foods. (Carbohydrates, starch, sugar are interchangeable terms because they are all converted to types of sugars in digestion. However we are distinguishing between carbohydrates and starches changed by manufacturing versus natural ones.) Therefore, manufactured starch and sugar will be limited to LTN, Little-To-No, status. However, you do not have to do without *natural* starch and sugar. This means that you will replace processed starch and sugar with natural milk and fruit sugars in the first phase of the diet. This will be easy to do and you will find you do not miss the refined, manufactured products at all. LTN, flour and white sugar products, then becomes dairy, fruit, vegetables, and natural carbs. *Natural Carbs* or *NC* are discussed more in Chapter 5. But first, we need to talk more about "real" and natural food vs. manufactured food.

But what is *real* food? *Natural* food? The distinctions blur in modern foods. We need to deconstruct modern foods and replace them with real foods in the mind. Therefore, we are going to categorize real food as the food our bodies can easily metabolize. This is food tracing back to the Agricultural Revolution and to ancient civilizations thousands of years ago as illustrated in the next chapter, Chapter 4, *Secret X Factor*.

4 SECRET X FACTOR
SSSA + **X**(NC + HP + NH + MC) = Fat Loss

So far, we've discussed the Starch and Sugar Addiction and the effects of industrial, processed foods. As stated before, however, this diet plan is a combination of powerful strategies at work. As a life source, food involves everything, such as intuition, love, passion, history, science, socialization, and culture. To emphasize one aspect over another results in lopsided, dieting failure.

The Secret X Factor is one of the most important parts of this diet. Though it is everywhere around us, it is a secret because we are unaware of its power. It has to do with metabolism and food choices and how some foods are not fattening simply because they are a part of metabolic history. Something great happens on this diet. That something great is that a *whole world of foods* is open to us, a whole world of delicious, satisfying, wonderful food that inherently does not cause weight gain, simply because it is natural to us and our bodies can metabolize it. This is in contrast to industrialized foods. Good metabolism does not require some secret plant from the tropics or a new pill but only the selection of the right foods based in ancient heritage.

The magic of our own bodies is full of mystery. Science cannot explain all the complexities, all the chemistry, that processes food into life energy. For understanding, we have to look at history. Ancient history. Why? Because our body metabolism, our body's nutritional needs, are based in prehistoric and ancient times in the foods people have eaten for many thousands of years. These foods are nutritious because they are part of the historic past and therefore essential for healthy metabolism. This includes foods from not only the hunting and gathering of the Stone Age cultures some 40,000 - 50,000 years ago, but those of the lush productive farming of the great agricultural civilizations over some 15,000 years ago. This is why your body can easily metabolize hefty natural carbs and bread as well as the traditional diet foods of meat and salads. But more on that later. For now, we need to focus on the tremendous variety of food choices we have for losing excess fat and for maintaining weight by eating according to our heritage. Otherwise, we will lose weight only to gain it back again.

That our bodies depend on a long past history of foods is shown in its nutritional needs. For example, the need for Vitamin C in citrus fruits and Vitamin D in sunshine didn't stop for people who migrated north to colder climates where fruit and sunshine were limited, causing scurvy and rickets. They still needed these nutrients. (Early Eskimos reportedly got vitamins such as C and D from eating organ meats of land and sea animals.)

The need for iodine in seafood is another good example, along with the health benefits of eating fish, even though we may live nowhere near an ocean. But our ancestors did. For thousands of years, people lived near oceans and tributary rivers for drinking water, irrigation, and food. The scenarios for the kinds of foods we need to eat are from the places where ancient civilizations thrived, in the warmer latitudes which provided a rich abundance of food. The areas around the Mediterranean are good examples as the originators of western civilizations and Eurasian cultures, where the peoples in Europe and Asia mixed and thrived before migration. This includes the earliest civilizations in Egypt along the mighty Nile, the earliest agricultural cities in Mesopotamia, the land between the rivers, the Tigris and Euphrates, as well as the classic Mediterranean cultures of Greece and Rome. Of course, civilizations were also thriving throughout Asia and in the Americas. All of the foods from all of these cultures are natural to us as preindustrial foods. However, emphasis is given to the Mediterranean areas as models and as progenitors to Western Civilization. (Asia and the Americas also provide us with some delicious foods for ancient metabolism and they too are included.) This is why the well-known Mediterranean Diet is effective. Because it involves *some* of these ancient foods. However, there are many more. These foods from long ago, our metabolic links to the past, include healthy fruits and vegetables so often missing in our own diets as well as a huge variety of other foods, in meat, dairy, beverages, breads, pastas, cereals, herbs, spices, nuts, and honey cakes -- all models for metabolic food choices.

If we look at a chart of time periods in technology, we can easily see that humans have not had time to adapt to an industrial diet of manufactured food. Technology characterizes the kinds of food we eat and the culture we live in. The Industrial Revolution, with machines and mass production factories began around 1760 with the mechanized spinning wheel in England, only some 250 years ago.

Technology Time Spans
40,000 Years

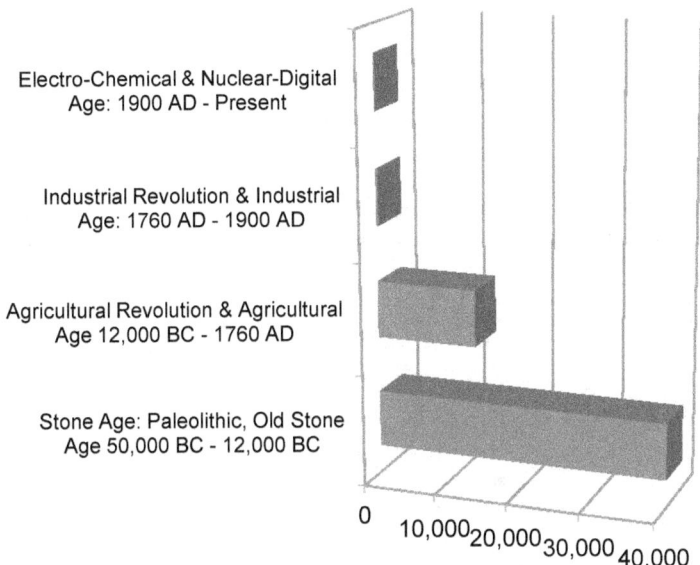

You will note on the chart that most of our past metabolic history is in the Stone Age and the Agricultural Age. The Industrial and Nuclear Digital Ages barely show up as a percentage in the past 40,000 years. (Scientists generally agree the human body has not changed for the last 40 to 45,000 years.) So what does it mean for the dieter? It means bread, pasta, and comfortable carbs along with other nutritious foods. The foods of the ages. On the chart, The Agricultural Age is roughly one fourth of the time period. This means, for example, cultivated grain products can be eaten for metabolic efficiency about a fourth of the time, as the diet will prove. To judge whether you can easily metabolize a food, ask yourself whether it is an ancient lands food or ancient food. Did the ancients eat the skins and seeds of fruits? Did they eat the skin of poultry? The fat? Of course. Since you are dieting to lose fat, however, you are limiting fat, but you can try a sample if you seem to want it. You'll realize how much you intuitively know about this and how it all comes together. Following are samples of the kinds of foods that are part of our healthy metabolism. The food lists are samples of the foods of the ages. The lists are not comprehensive but indicate the tremendous variety of foods we can eat for dieting - the kinds of foods that are inherited for efficient metabolism.

Food History

Prehistoric and ancient dates are estimates as changes were gradual over thousands of years.

Dates also vary with sources consulted. In tracing our food metabolism history, change is to be considered additive and each age includes all of the foods before. Lists of ancient foods are those in archeological records and are not intended to be all-inclusive but to provide a general overview.

Last Great Ice Age, the Pleistocene – 1 million BC to 18,000-12,000 BC. Icy tundra covered Europe and China. Climate then warms to that similar to today. The end of the Ice Age allowed agriculture to flourish in ancient civilizations and spread throughout Europe and Asia.

Early Peoples
? – 60,000 BC
Tropical to
sub-tropical latitudes -
coasts & waterways

fruits
nuts
seeds
leafy greens
roots
fish
shellfish
water birds
eggs
wild game

Old Stone Age
100,000 BC – 12,000 BC

Ice Age
(Europe, China)
Seasonal –
woods, plateaus,
mountains
fruits, berries
nuts
seeds
roots
fish
birds
eggs
wild game such
as pigs,
  goats, sheep

New Stone Age
12,000 BC–4,000 BC
Village Life – More tools
& Crafts
Beginnings of Agriculture
15,000 BC - 11,000 BC

Agricultural Revolution
9,000 BC – 2,000 BC
cultivated crops
domesticated
animals
wild wheat and
barley
cereals
roots, tubers
wild pears
nuts: wild
acorns,
almonds,
pistachios

By 5,000 BC:
Wheat and barley
cultivated in
Southeastern
Europe, Egypt,
Turkey, Caucasus,
Iran, India. Rice
and millet grown in
China and
Southeast Asia.

Mesopotamia
Mesopotamia cultivates the first wheat and barley from wild strains – 11,000 BC.

fish	onions	pears
mutton	garlic	apricots
pork	leeks	pomegranates
ducks	cucumbers	nuts
pigeons	cress	pistachio nuts
wheat	mustard	milk
millet	herbs	cheese
barley	lettuce	butter
barley ale	grapes	vegetable oils
(1 gal/day)	raisins	honey
chickpeas	dates	cake (flour, eggs, milk,
lentils	figs	honey)
beans	plums	flatbread (unleavened
	apples	bread)

Ancient Egypt
15,000 BC – 2,400 BC

15,000-10,000 BC	5,200 BC	3,000 – 2,400 BC
antelope	cattle	water birds & their eggs
hippos	pigs	pigeons
fish	sheep	ducks
shellfish	goats	crane
geese	cultivated emmer wheat	small uncooked,
ducks	barley	salted, pickled birds and
	cultivated flax (ropes,	fish
	clothing)	beef
		grapes
		figs
		berries
		onions
		milk
		cheese
		wine – red/
		beer/ale
		flat bread
		yeast bread
		pastries
		sweet cakes

The Egyptians developed enclosed ovens for baking yeast-leavened bread from wild yeasts in 3,000 BC. Egyptian food feasts included over 40 different kinds of breads and pastries, both raised and flat, made from flour and various ingredients including honey, milk, and eggs. The Commoner's daily food however is thought to have been a mainstay of flatbread, ale, and onions.

Ancient Greece
800 BC – 150 BC

Milk used for cheese
rather than drinking.
 Breakfasts were bread
and wine.
 Dinner was the large
meal of the day.
 Ate with hands, few
utensils.

fish
shellfish
wild game
birds
chicken
lamb
beef
pork
pomegranates
apples

beans
peas
chickpeas (garbanzo
beans0
lentils
grains
barley, wheat
bread
cheese
eggs
milk
olive oil
vinegar
grapes
figs
herbs
nuts
asparagus
nuts

asparagus
artichokes
cabbage
olives
pears
plums
squash
leeks
radishes
turnips
wild celery
cress
Romaine lettuce
carrots
cucumber
wine
honey mead
beer

Ancient Rome
100 BC – 500 AD

Similar to that of Ancient
Greece.
Breakfast was often bread
dipped in olive oil with
wine.
Dinner was the large
meal of the day. Ate
mostly with hands.
Utensils used for serving.
Milk was used for making
cheese rather than
drinking.

eggs
bread
cereal
cheese

fish
shellfish
game
domestic fowl
pork
figs
dates
nuts
apples
pears
grapes
cabbage
parsnips
lettuce/salad/romaine

asparagus
onion
garlic
radishes
lentils
beans
beets
herbs
spices
cakes, pastries
    sweetened w/honey
pancakes
wine

Flour & Sugar
Age of Agriculture

Flour

Both white and brown flour are produced. White bread is eaten mostly by the rich as it is more expensive, taking longer to produce.

Sugarcane from India

Darius of Persia and his soldiers saw sugar cane growing in India and called it the reed that produces honey without bees. 510 BC. Ancients used mostly honey and fruit sugars for sweetening.

Ancient Americas, Tropical Islands, Asia
Time frames vary. List is example only.

Indigenous meats, game, fish, birds, seafood.	yams	tea
maize/corn	sweet potatoes	noodles
tortilla/taco	potatoes	rice
tamale	grapefruit	millet
pineapple	bell peppers	soy sauce
papaya	chili peppers	tofu
banana	winter & summer squash	sesame seeds/oil
avocado	pumpkin	bamboo shoots
tomatoes	beans-pinto, red, black	sake/rice wine
cacao	vanilla bean	herbs
coffee	peanuts	spices

European Medieval Food
1100 – 1500 AD

	barley bread, cereal	cabbage
Increased	barley ale	leeks
emphasis on	French wine	spinach
meat and bread	cheese	parsley
as foundation	milk	onions
foods with	eggs	garlic
fewer fruits and	salted and preserved for	honey
vegetables in the	winter	sugar, spices – imported
colder climates.	fish, beef, pork	
beef		
pork		
lamb		
fish		
birds		

Industrial Revolution
1760 – 2000 AD

Increasing mass production of foods	refined	chemicals
Refined flours	processed	artificial flavors, colors
Refined white sugar from sugar beets and sugar cane	treated	preservatives
	cloned, hybrid	starchy fillers
	frozen, boxed, canned, shaped, formed, wrapped	corn syrup
		salt, excessive
1700's – Wheat replaces rye and barley as primary grain in Europe when sturdier wheat is developed for the colder climate	.	sugar, excessive
		hydrogenated fats

The X Factor is the foundation behind your diet, the secret to not only losing excess weight but keeping it off. In choosing to eat the natural foods, the real foods, the preindustrial foods, you are choosing the kinds of foods your body can metabolize easily, the foods your ancestors and all of humankind ate for thousands of years. Most importantly, your food choices open up to a whole new world of delicious foods beyond traditional dieting.

Food is the product of technology and culture.

The ancients, the Greeks and Romans, did not drink much milk because they did not have ice and refrigeration readily available for preservation, though they would sometimes get snow and ice from the mountains. But they made cheese, such as goat cheese, and cheese was a big part of the diet. In other words, milk and dairy products are ancient real foods.

Ancient peoples did not eat much beef because they used cattle for working. They also had to live near waterways of rivers and oceans. Consequently, fresh and saltwater fish and fowl are more ancient foods than beef. You will note on your diet that they are more efficient for metabolism. However, red meat is still a natural ancient food from wild game and domesticated animals.

The food in Europe during castle days, is not fully representative of the source food, the foods of ancient times. Foods of northern peoples, such as those of medieval Europeans, lacked the abundance of fruits and vegetables available in warmer climates. As we inherited their food patterns culturally, the European cold weather foods of meat and bread still characterize popular food choices of today such as fast food hamburgers. Why are so many in our culture obese and still gaining? We find that what has not been revealed through science can be discovered through history. The lists of the foods of ancient civilizations explains metabolic heritage, as the body knows how to metabolize them and use them for food. This adds up to a whole treasure chest of food choices as well as to generous servings of foods easily used by the body without weight gain.

This also means that we can eat all kinds of natural carbs and preindustrial breads and pastas without weight gain. This is further explored in the next chapter, *Natural Carbs*.

5 NATURAL CARBS

SSSA + X(**NC** + HP + NH + MC) = Fat Loss

We hear all the time that we need to eat natural foods and eat more fruits and vegetables. Then we are told that carbohydrates are bad and we must limit them to lose weight. Diet books and diet plans count carbs rather than calories. Meanwhile, what's natural becomes a blur beyond raw produce, especially for young people, who have grown up eating convenience supermarket foods and fast foods with little knowledge of nutrition beyond the phrase "healthy food." They know healthy food is better but cannot explain what or why and have little interest in changing the food they enjoy, indeed have learned to rely on, for sustenance. Small wonder, as it is all a muddle of food in disguise. Some of us seek organic food as a ready answer to escape the chemical food industry while starch and sugar addicts tune in to nonfat-everything-sugar's-okay. Meanwhile, the whole country, is increasingly becoming obese in staggeringly record numbers.

The dilemma is not easy. The culprits are tricky. A strategy of defense is required. Yet, the study and planning for delicious, healthy, nonfattening food is a challenge, requiring some effort and time. Most people look to sundry diet plans, infomercial contraptions, the media, and advertising for answers with little lasting success beyond yoyo-ing with lose-and-gain, lose-and-gain. You are fortunate to have found *Love Your Diet*, with comfortable, self-loving diet plans. The reasoning and strategy have been done for you. All you have to do is put it to work.

First of all, carbs are not bad. We need them. To severely limit them is a threat to well-being and health. And those experienced with the carb-limiting, carb-counting dieting will attest to the torture of hunger and cravings, as the body cries out for what it needs. Some dieters, probably friends of yours, have even gotten serious illnesses after going on these kinds of diets. The key is *natural* carbs. Carb tricks involves exchanging the bad carbs with all the carbohydrates the ancients ate, including heavy duty carbs like beans, rice, and potatoes and of course, the fruits and vegetables so familiar to the dieter. As we've learned from looking at historical foods, our bodies need all the nutrients from the Age of Agriculture's variety of cultivated rich grains, vegetables, fruit, and dairy foods, as well as from the Stone Age wild game, fish, greens, berries, seeds, nuts, and tubers (tubers are root foods such as potatoes). Breads and pastas are included. Again, most diets emphasize Stone Age type eating, too rigorous and sparse, leading to long-term failure. This one celebrates the best of food, which has to include the abundance of farming and agriculture, an important part of our natural metabolic food heritage.

Of course, the ancient food model doesn't mean you need to grind your own grain, just as modern Stone Age type diets don't require a hunting and gathering trip to the wild. It means that flour and whole grains are foods natural to our metabolism.

We must also pause and give credit to all the science and technology that is feeding many millions of people with mass-produced foods and successful crops. Without mass production to market, we could not feed everyone. However, we must look at the problems that are causing excessive fat as the press of world populations create decline in the quality of available foods.

SSSA – Stop Starch and Sugar Addiction with Natural Carbohydrates

Natural Carbs. This is the key to stopping starch and sugar addiction. To stop this addiction, you need to limit refined white sugar and other overly-processed manufactured foods produced and packaged in factories. In the diet menus, you will be replacing refined white sugar, which is highly concentrated and stripped of metabolic nutrients, with natural raw sugars, raw honey, and natural maple syrup. (Honey has been on the planet for millions of years and is a very ancient food.) Even refined white sugar can be tolerated in small amounts. But with processed foods, you are talking a huge amount of sugar and syrup that disrupt metabolism and add fat. To stop the addiction, you will be replacing refined white sugar and manufactured starch with *natural* milk sugars and *natural* fruit sugars. The first three to four days of the diet remarkably easily stop this addiction.

As discussed earlier, all carbohydrates are converted from

starch into different sugars that can be utilized by the body. This is what makes a discussion of carbohydrates so confusing. However, the working confusion is resolved with the replacement of *disguised* manufactured starch and sugar with the *natural* starch and sugar in real foods.

Think about what you eat to keep the excess fat on with a minimum of effort: constant snacks, constant refined white sugar (cookies, cake, candy), and fast food (most fast food chains are using the same types of manufactured products as on the store shelves). These are the foods feeding your addiction without satisfying your hunger. You have to say to yourself that these foods are addictive, for whatever reason. So to be serious about weight loss, you have to restrict your intake of these foods and *replace* them with the foods your body needs for metabolism.

This is dramatically illustrated in the first stages of this diet. The starter menus restrict the foods causing the addiction and replace them with natural starch and sugar. You will not believe how great you will feel within the first three days as your body begins to hum with the starch and sugar it needs. So this is the key: you are stopping starch and sugar addiction, not starch and sugar. Natural starch and sugar are needed by your body.

Frequently on diets, because of the starch and sugar addiction, people fool themselves and think that it is good to eat manufactured foods that are "made from *natural* ingredients." They eat nibble snacks such as chips and whole grain crackers thinking this is healthy eating without all the sweet sugar. Or, they go ahead and eat the refined starch and sugar foods, thinking *nonfat everything* is alright. The truth is your body needs a little fat for digestion, such as to help metabolize the fat-soluble vitamins, A, D, E, and K. The truth is that for a multitude of reasons, manufactured shelf products distort the body's need for natural foods. The truth is that refined white sugar is not a natural food and is full of addiction, especially as used in factory foods. Natural sugars, honey, raw sugar, milk products, fruit do not cause this addiction. But it is not just the sugar. Manufactured products have excessive starch as fillers in the food to make it more profitable, along with corn syrup, salt, fat, and flavorings which serve to trick the taste buds and impersonate real food. So in addition to the concentrated white sugar, other sources of addiction are all the added chemicals, colorings, flavorings, and so on. We've discussed it before, but this cannot be emphasized enough if you want to lose weight. The addiction is caused by your body trying to get the nutrients it needs to metabolize the food. There is no coding for the strange new food. As mentioned earlier, the body stores all the extra "food" as fat to *try* to deal with later, just as you store all your junk to deal with later.

Potatoes - Potato Chips

Consider the distortion of potato chips, which seem like a healthy snack made of a natural food, potatoes. (Please note that other manufactured snack foods contain this distortion. Potato chips are used only as an example.) Let's compare potato chips with real potatoes. First of all, potatoes are alive with nutrients. Left in the cupboard too long, they will grow shoots and roots. Placed on a window sill in water, a potato will grow into a leafy potato plant. Potatoes are alive and full of nutrients. Potato chips will never grow into a plant, but will only grow rubbery and stale. Potato chips are not potatoes.

Consider the following comparisons:

Potato chips are marketed in bright shiny vacuum-packed packages listing a multitude of exciting flavorings from cheddar sour cream to smoky mesquite barbeque. Just open the bag and eat. Potatoes are in the produce section as modest lumpy veggies in various shades of brown that have to be washed and cooked.

Calories: You would have to eat over *five* big 10-ounce potatoes at around 300 calories each to equal the 1500 calories in 10 ounces of potato chips.

Carbohydrate: You would have to eat two and a half large potatoes at 60 grams of carbohydrate to equal the 150 grams in 10 ounces of potato chips.

Fat: With the potato at .28 natural grams of fat, you would have to eat 357, 10-ounce potatoes, or 223 pounds, to equal the 100 grams of fat in the potato chips. Adding butter or sour cream to the 10-ounce potato would require two cups of sour cream (1 cup = 48 grams fat) or eight tablespoons butter (1 tablespoon = 12 grams of fat).

Salt: The sodium or salt in the potato chip exceeds that in the potato by more than 100 times. Adding your own salt and a tablespoon of sour cream still leaves the potato chips ahead with four times the salt as shown in the following table comparing just one ounce of potato chips.

Sodium (Salt) Content
Recommended Daily Levels of Sodium:
AI (Adequate Intake) - 1500 mg. (milligrams)
UL (Upper Level) - 2300 mg.

1 ounce potato chips	1,684 mg sodium
10 ounce white potato	14 mg sodium
1/8 teaspoon salt	290 mg sodium
1 tablespoon nonfat sour cream	23 mg.sodium

Eating just a small three-ounce bag of potato chips at 5052 mg sodium far exceeds the upper level recommendation of 2300 mg daily.

The excessive salt in manufactured foods greatly contributes to water retention and mineral imbalances that can affect your metabolism. You are very thirsty after eating them because of all the salt. Most manufactured foods have excessive salt added for flavor. Whenever you mix or put together your own natural foods and seasonings, you are ingesting less salt. Natural foods already contain salt on their own. Add herbs and spices for flavoring in place of salt. Herbs and spices are gifts of the earth, little gifts of the gods, for food pleasure. As well as providing taste sensation, herbs and spices contain small amounts of plant nutrients that feed metabolism. See the table at the end of the chapter for a comparison of salt with herbs and spices.

When you compare a list of ingredients in a potato to that of potato chips, for the potato you will see a list of nutrients, such as carbohydrate count, protein, fat, vitamins and minerals; in the potato chips you will see nutrients (many as a result of added *whey*, a milk byproduct of cheese making) *and* a host of other strange ingredients, including preservatives, colorings, and flavorings which are not part of the natural food. The chart below lists comparisons between potatoes and potato chips. Sweet potatoes and yams are included as part of the diet as options because they are very rich in Vitamin A. Vitamin A, produced naturally from carotene in food, is a fat-soluble antioxidant vitamin that fights disease, nourishes the skin and eyes, and replenishes surface membranes inside the body. Here are some of the extra ingredients in the potato chips not found in a potato: hydrolyzed corn protein, corn and/or cottonseed oil, monosodium glutamate, natural and artificial flavors, sugar dextrose, corn flour, corn starch, disodium phosphate, artificial colors, yellow 6 Lake, yellow 6, yellow 5, red 40, yellow 5 Lake, blue 1 Lake, blue 1.

In a comparison of white potato to potato chips, calorie by calorie, the potato, with sour cream added to make up the essential amino acid methionine and B2 riboflavin, has one to four times the nutrients of the potato chips, which already have a milk product, whey, added.

Again, this is more than about potato chips; they are used here as an example of manufactured, packaged foods. Read the labels.

In summary, on this diet, you will view starch and sugar addiction as an effect of the foods you eat which are high in refined white sugar, corn syrup, added starch, excessive salt, excessive fat, and chemicals for preservation, leavening, coloring, and flavoring. The menus will show you how.

Bread and Pasta – Natural Carbs

Bread, the staff of life, and all grain products are very ancient foods. So it follows that we should be able to metabolize them efficiently. This is quite true when we stick to the natural and whole grain products. Bread that has been preserved and overly processed for shelf life is sure to help pack on pounds. However, using ancient foods as a guide, you will find the uses of grains and breads, following the evolution of their use, can be used without weight gain. This includes fresh bakery bread without preservatives.

First, however, we must discuss leavenings, the yeast and other ingredients used to raise bread products. Yeast is a very ancient living food used to ferment grains and fruits for alcoholic beverages and to make bread for many thousands of years and is therefore compatible with the body. This is the reason for its mouth-watering metabolic invitation. However, leavening agents such as baking powder and baking soda are often made using sodium aluminum sulfate and sodium aluminum phosphate. This puts them in a category of industrialized foods unfamiliar to metabolism. However, cream of tartar, when used in place of these products, is compatible as a byproduct of wine making. More experimentation is needed as to whether cream of tartar leavened products are metabolized cleanly without weight gain. However, manufactured foods contain the chemical kinds which make them fat producers. This is why foods leavened with baking powder and baking soda should be used sparingly, if at all, especially while dieting. This includes all cake-type products such as biscuits, muffins, scones, cookies, and cakes. Using the food of the ages as a guide, the list of grain products from least fattening to most fattening would look like the following table.

Bread & Grain Products
Rated Best to Worst for Metabolic Compatibility as Natural Real Foods Determined by Use in History

Best: Least Fat Effect

Rating	Product Today	Reason
1	Whole grain cereals, to cook. Whole wheat, barley, flax, brown rice, rye, oatmeal.	Stone Age – 50,000 BC to 12,000 BC Gathered Seeds including wild wheat and barley. Wheat was emmer wheat, a crude wild wheat gathered in Mediterranean areas. Wild rice in Asia. Whole grain natural nutrients. Often mixed with vegetable soups and sometimes eaten mixed with water or milk as a drinkable cereal or gruel.
2	Whole grain flatbreads and pastas without leavening. Pita, tortillas, pasta (no baking powder, baking soda, preservatives, trans fats, or other additives).	Emmer wheat and barley are cultivated into domestic strains. 11,000 BC. Beginnings of Agricultural Revolution. First breads are ground, mixed with water or fruit juice and cooked. Whole grain natural nutrients.
3	Yeast leavened bread, whole wheat. Yeast is ancient and compatible. Home baked or fresh bakery bread without preservatives or additives. Whole wheat french bread.	3,000 BC: Egyptians bake yeast breads from wild yeasts. Northern Europeans and those in British Isles also baked bread from wild yeast very early.
4	Yeast leavened bread, white, enriched. Includes french bread and pizza crust. Without preservatives or additives.	Both dark and light breads are eaten, with the rich preferring white, but

	Pasta, white, enriched, nonleavened, usually preferred with white flour.	more expensive to produce. White has fewer nutrients with wheat germ and seed coat removed. Romans. 100 BC – 500 AD
5	Pastry without leavening. Pie crust	Pastry is unleavened flour product but usually high in fats and sugar and usually made with less-nutritious white flour.
6	Pastry, yeast-leavened. Donuts, rolls, maple bars, etc. Fresh baked, no preservatives.	Yeast leavening is metabolic complement. However, today's fat and high refined sugar content require restraint.

Worst: Most Fat Effect

7	Tea breads, biscuits, scones, cookies, cake donuts, cakes, pancakes leavened with chemical baking powder and baking soda.	Baking powder and baking soda are relatively new leavening agents, the products of the manufacturing age since 1800s. Leavened with eggs okay. Home baked borderline okay. Usually high sugar and fat content.
8	Off the shelf flour products: cookies, cakes, muffins, crackers, donuts, rolls, bread, chips, cereals. Manufactured, processed, preserved.	Industrial. Last 200 years. Packed with artificial ingredients.

Applying the fundamentals in this chart in choosing natural real grains and avoiding additives, preservatives, and products made with baking powder and baking soda, you will find you can enjoy bread and pasta without weight gain, especially if used moderately. *However, this is only true if you are also restricting refined white sugar and using natural sugars* such as honey, raw sugar, demerara, and natural maple syrup. If you *continually* eat the bad carbs, the addictive manufactured starch and sugar we've been discussing, *you will continue to gain weight no matter what the rest of your diet*. After you've stopped the addiction, you can get away with infrequent use of these foods. However, you will find you do not miss them at all as you replace them with delicious more natural carbs Recommended is to get a bread machine and make your own bread. That way you are sure of the ingredients. A bread machine is easy to use, keeps the kitchen clean, comes with a lot of recipes, and makes great bread.

6 HIGH PROTEIN

SSSA + X(NC + **HP** + NH + MC) = Fat Loss

Protein is so important because it plays so many roles. Protein builds, repairs, and replaces all the cells in the body such as tissues, hair, skin, muscles, and organs. It is a part of every cell and necessary for health and vitality. Protein is necessary for the metabolism taking place inside the cells. Having enough protein during dieting also helps control hunger, prevent fatigue, and maintain skin tone during fat loss.

In digestion, protein is broken down into amino acids. There are some 22 amino acids but not all of them can be produced by the body. There are 8 Essential Amino Acids, or EAAs, that must be provided daily by the diet. Since all these amino acids depend on each other, without the EAA's, protein cannot be utilized. In this case, the incomplete protein is stored in the body as carbohydrate glucose. You can readily see that inadequate protein contributes to excess fat because it is not metabolized. Complete proteins however are lean nutrients building cells, skin, and muscles.

The foods that supply the eight essential amino acids are called *complete* protein foods. Other foods have protein too, such as fruits and vegetables. However, they are not complete proteins as they do not provide adequate amounts. For example, beans have high amounts of protein but they are not complete proteins by themselves because other foods are needed to boost some of their low amino acids. Soybeans are an exception as a plant and are classified as a complete protein. Fruits and vegetables have all kinds of little amounts of protein to contribute to the EAA foods, adding to efficient metabolism of other foods, but again, are not complete proteins.

Foods that have complete proteins are meat, poultry, fish, eggs, milk, and other dairy products (and soybeans). To ensure adequate amounts, some of these complete protein foods must be eaten daily. Of the three food groups (protein, carbohydrates, fats), protein is the most difficult to maintain in adequate amounts. Therefore, protein levels get special attention.

How much protein do you need? The National Research

Council of the National Academy of Sciences sets Recommended Dietary Allowances, RDAs, for nutrients (See RDAs in *Love Your Diet Vitamins and Minerals.* The daily amount for protein should be about half your body weight in grams of protein. However, the body weight should be your target weight, or what you should weigh, to be within a normal weight range. So for a target weight of 190 pounds, around 80 grams of protein, more or less, are needed each day.

You'll see that getting enough protein takes some attention and planning. The menu guides provide for protein levels around 20 grams each for breakfast, lunch, and dinner with additional protein in snacks. These protein levels are maintained with foods that are complete proteins in eggs, dairy and meat products. All the nutritious fresh fruits and vegetables you'll be eating will also be adding contributing, if not complete, protein. Protein amounts for all the diet foods are listed in the paper-printed version of *Calorie Counter* in the Love Your Diet book series.

Breakfast protein is very important in laying the foundation for the day in preventing hunger and fatigue while dieting. Therefore make an extra effort to get 15 to 20 grams of protein for breakfast. A cup of milk is about 8 grams protein. An egg has about 6 grams. Eggs are a popular breakfast food with good protein and packed with enough nutrients to produce a whole chicken. They include the fat-soluble vitamins A, D, and E. Eggs are also a very real and ancient food, as people gathered the eggs of water birds to eat. However eggs are also high in cholesterol at some 200 mg (and lecithin, which helps metabolize cholesterol) and some recommendations are for only one egg a day, though many health enthusiasts eat eggs. Eggs are a favorite of nutritionists and body trainers because they provide protein and are easy, nutritious, and economical. The whites of eggs have no cholesterol and are high in protein so that if you are concerned with cholesterol experiment in eating only one egg with yolk and more whites, though the yolks are more nutritious and tasty. There are also lower-cholesterol, more-expensive eggs on the market with only 180 mg per egg. However, research continues as to how much foods, including eggs, cause bad cholesterol. Using lowfat dairy products also reduce cholesterol as well as fat intake. Note that nonfat products have very little if any Vitamin A, a fat-soluble vitamin. This is why lowfat is preferable to nonfat. The body needs some fat to synthesize oil-soluble vitamins, digest food, and to keep skin, hair, and tissues healthy. (Note how extremely lowfat diets are drying to skin and hair, while the overweight frequently have nice skin without wrinkles. The excess body fat however has health and quality of life issues. The point is that some dietary fat is needed.)

One half cup milk on cereal (4 grams) and one egg (6 grams) still equal only about 10 grams complete protein for breakfast. Something more is needed to make the amount closer to 20 grams. Unless you find lean meat for breakfast palatable and convenient, which can cover all the protein needed, another protein food must be added. More eggs, a half cup of cottage cheese, or one cup yogurt, or a high protein nutrition drink round out the needed protein amount.

Cottage cheese is very high in protein at about 25-28 grams per cup (8 ounces) and therefore always a good protein food. As a matter of interest, cottage cheese has more protein but less than half the calcium of milk or yogurt: 1 cup 1% cottage cheese, 138 mg calcium; lowfat yogurt, 448 mg calcium; 1% milk, 305 mg calcium. Therefore using a variety of these foods provides balance.

High protein nutrition and diet drinks are very convenient protein boosters. These are based in soybean or whey (milk byproduct of cheese making) and vary as to taste and cost. Experiment to find your favorite most affordable drink by purchasing small amounts of different kinds. Used frequently, the good tasting ones can still be expensive so they are best as supplements to other foods. Read the labels for protein and sugar content. You may also find you get hungry much faster when drinking only liquid protein drinks. Adding solid food, such as fruit or yogurt makes the liquid drink more satisfying for a longer period of time. In addition, you can make your own high-protein drink by adding dry milk to regular milk and thereby increasing protein and all nutrients. The flavor may not be that good however, but you can experiment with adding one tablespoon flavoring such as honey or chocolate syrup.

Yogurt

Yogurt has a very prominent place in the diet because it is nutritious, provides protein at low cost, and is very convenient, especially during the day when you are on the go. Forms of yogurt, some as liquid, like kefir, have been a food for at least 5,000 years. Yogurt is milk cultured with *Lactobacillus acidophilus* and other cultures such as *L. bulgaricus, S. thermophilus, L.casei, R. rhamnosus, and B.bifidum.* (The complete names are very long.) The bacteria are healthy stimulation to the body's intestinal bacteria, a necessary and normal part of digestion and metabolism. They help the intestines interact with digestive enzymes to manufacture B vitamins. Poor diets and antibiotics can deplete these bacteria. Yogurt therefore not only provides B-complex vitamins but helps replenish and boost synthesis of B vitamins in the body.

The use of yogurt along with other dairy foods provides nerve-building nutrients such as calcium, magnesium, potassium, and the B vitamins, all of which contribute to the calm nerves and tranquil feelings on the diet.

As emphasized previously however, do *not* eat yogurt that is packed with sugar to attract consumers with over 200 calories. Eat the low calorie at 100 to 120 calories, which is yogurt artificially sweetened and flavored. This can also be mixed with fully natural yogurt to get both worlds of health and taste. We'll refer to this mixed yogurt as Love Your Diet or LYD yogurt. Fresh fruit such as dark cherries, berries, and blueberries round out a tasty, very nutritious satisfying food. You may also want to try kefir, a liquid yogurt-like, buttermilk-tasting, product enthusiasts say is even more healthy than yogurt. Popular in Europe, it can also now be found in smaller US towns.

Meats

Of course meat is the classic provider of protein. All types of meat (beef, pork, poultry, fish, shellfish) are high in protein and provide at least 20 grams for an average serving of 3 to 4 ounces. However, fresh meat foods are not always convenient throughout the day. The use of milk products to supply the needed protein is a more convenient and less expensive way to maintain these levels. However, when reducing fat, it makes sense to limit fats, so choose lowfat milk products. Read the labels. As mentioned earlier, nonfat products do not have any Vitamin A.

As for preserved meats, you will need to limit these while dieting because they have chemical preservatives inhibiting to metabolism. This includes cold cuts, ham, bacon, sausage, hot dogs, and sliced deli meats. As for the fat and skins of meats, ask yourself if the ancient ancestors ate them. Of course they did. However, since you are reducing fat, it makes sense to limit fat, so keep fat to a minimum by only sampling that extra meat and poultry fat. And of course, coldwater fish oil, as omega 3, is very much recommended now.

Some may wonder, upon reflection, why we need to eat meat at all. The answer is in our cells, in our genes, in our ancient heritage. Our bodies genetically call for meat. However, it is very ecologically expensive to provide food for livestock that in turn provide meat. As we consider the world's billions of humans eating meat, the future may demand alternatives for protein that are more sustainable. Currently, dairy products, soybeans, and sea farming offer options.

Fats and Oils

Fats and oils are not treated separately as they are very much a part of the diet but limited by calories and type. Fats are of three categories: saturated, monounsaturated, and polyunsaturated. Saturated fats are solid at room temperature and represent animal fat and processed vegetable fats made solid in manufacturing, such as in shortening and some margarines. Monounsaturated and polyunsaturated fats are vegetable fats that remain liquid at room temperature. Paradoxically, the polyunsaturated vegetable oils so promoted in earlier decades have been determined to be a threat to cardiovascular health when used extensively by themselves. These are the omega 6 type fats in most vegetable oils. The missing ingredient is omega 3 type fats, which must be balanced with omega 6 fats to be healthy. Omega 3 fats are found in cold water fish oils, flaxseed, and canola oil. Soybean oil also has some omega 3. Monounsaturated fats are in a separate category and regarded as safe. Olive oil is a monounsaturated fat. (Note that olive oil is an ancient link food as is flax, an ancient source for food and clothing.) In the diet, the cold pressed, first press olive oil should be used as it is the most natural and nutritious. Because of the omega 6 scare, butter is back in favor. Butter is an animal fat and a saturated fat, but can be used sparingly. Butter is an ancient link real food. Fats and oils are high calorie at 100 calories per tablespoon so of course their excessive use in manufactured foods, along with all the other ingredients in processing, add to the starch and sugar weight gain.

Balanced nutrition in the real foods, including protein and fat, is important for health and metabolism. In the next chapter are reasons why considering hunger itself must be a part of successful dieting.

7 NO HUNGER

$$SSSA + X(NC + HP + \mathbf{NH} + MC) = Fat\ Loss$$

The body fights back when weight is reduced by extreme diets using hunger and unbalanced foods The body experiences these kinds of weight loss as a threat to survival, as a survival test. When the dieting is over, the body immediately adds the weight back to its former level of comfort, as protection against the next dangerous assault.

This is why you must lose excess fat without hunger, without threat, without stress, to the body. The body must feel it is safe to "let go" of excessive fat, to let down defenses towards losing weight. To ignore this is to fail to maintain weight loss and to have to repeat dieting over and over. For successful weight loss, you must avoid hunger and its stress to the body.

However, the hunger to avoid is of two kinds. The first kind is the feelings of hunger we get when the body feels the need for food. The other kind of hunger, the *hidden hunger*, is when the body is not getting the right balance of foods for proper metabolism. These foods are the variety of natural real foods to which the body has needed for many thousands of years. Both of these kinds of hunger create stress to the body, finally resulting in weight gain, not weight loss. These two kinds of hunger are interrelated in our past. First, let's see how to avoid the more obvious feelings of hunger.

Hunger Torture

Hunger is torture. That's why the feeling is called hunger *pains*, as the body signals with need that it's time to eat. Denying hunger is as impossible as denying the need to urinate. Yet hunger is a necessary part of most diet plans, treated as though it doesn't matter much or that it is an unstated punishment for greed. Well it does matter. It matters a lot. And the hunger-sin theme beats the dieter over the head with inferiority, inadequacy, and at most martyrdom in feelings of fasting. Diets of hunger are culprits and to promote them should be unacceptable. Imagine trying to force the biology of the body to deny the need to urinate. The attempt would lead to health problems and to medical and emotional disorders, just as it does with extreme dieting.

On this diet plan, you are not to go hungry. When you feel hungry, eat. Continue to eat the *natural real* foods. Eat as many fruits and vegetables as you want. Eat as much yogurt as you want. As much meat, and so on. But you will be staying within some minimal guidelines, discussed later, that will prevent hunger while losing excess fat.

Hunger is your body's way of saying it needs food. Once feelings of hunger begin, they do not go away, but continue to increase. Hunger feelings therefore go through different stages or levels:

> *Level 1 Hunger* is felt as very slight twinges or interrupted reminders that you will need to eat soon. Level 1 hunger can be forgotten for small amounts of time.
> *Level 2 Hunger* is more persistent and does not go away. You feel full-blown hunger and want to eat.
> *Level 3 Hunger* is very strong and powerful. At Level 3, you feel as though you are starving and must eat immediately!

Level 3 hunger is to be avoided. At Level 3, you are vulnerable to eating any food available. Level 3 is the starvation level, the point at which your body signals frantically that it must have food to survive. Of course, you know it has plenty of fat stores to use and is not starving. On other diets, which require enduring this starvation level, you are well acquainted with the mighty Level 3 hunger pangs! Only sheer will power can endure them and then only for so long. After a week of intermittent Level 3 hunger, the diet is usually broken by even the strongest-willed who succumb to the most outrageously fat food they can find.

On this diet, you must eat at Level 1 hunger. You know that real hunger, once it begins, is only going to increase until you eat. Satisfying the first feelings of hunger assures your body that it is not starving and can relax in the security of food. The body will only fight back when it feels deprived of food. Body metabolism will slow down and once food is available, the body will want to consume voraciously and put the fat, the security, back in place. This is only natural. Therefore, on this diet you must avoid hunger and its stress on the body.

Hidden Hunger

Many of us may find it difficult to imagine a time when food is scarce to nonexistent. That's why we may think hunger is more a state of mind than a biological force, especially for the overweight. But when we consider that for many thousands of years ancestors had to survive during extended periods without enough food, we can see how our bodies are programmed to protect against starvation. To the body, constant hunger signals the threat of starvation, regardless of weight or fat stores. The body remembers the famines of the past. Our conscious minds do not.

The instinct to fight hunger is a basic survival response that predates history. In the Old Stone Age, in hunting and gathering cultures, constant movement was necessary to find food. It was a full time endeavor. The restlessness of the hunt and constant foraging for plants were pushed by the stress of hunger. Satisfying that hunger assured survival. The foods that nourished and comforted the body were wild game and plants. Food had to supply energy for hunting and gathering as well as for body warmth during the Ice Age. The high protein diet of meat provided the muscle strength for the bursts of physical exertion needed by the carnivorous diet while the hides provided clothing and shelter to survive danger and exposure.

The Old Stone Age with its constant search for food was left far behind at the end of the last great Ice Age around 18,000 BC to 12,000 BC. In the warmer climate, in regions closer to the equator, plants and animals flourished and people began to live in small villages marking the beginning of the New Stone Age or Neolithic revolution. See Chapter 4 tables on the Stone Age and Agricultural Civilizations. (There are people in the world today still living in hunting gathering cultures, mostly in isolated areas and warmer climates that can support this way of life. These people are also linked genetically to common origins. See Spencer Wells, *The Journey of Man.)*

From these early beginnings, the New Stone Age continued for thousands of years and change was gradual. People in permanent villages began to grow crops and domesticate animals, the beginning of the Agricultural Revolution. Wild wheat and barley, gathered and stored in 15,000 BC were first cultivated in 11,000 BC.

Animals domesticated from 11,000 – 6,000 BC were sheep, goats, cattle, and donkeys along with companion pets. Dogs were domesticated from wild wolves by 11,000 BC and cats from wildcats by 7,000 BC; dogs were hunters and protectors while the cats kept rodents away.

By 5,000 BC, wheat and barley were grown in Egypt, Turkey, southeastern Europe, the Caucasus, Iran, and India. At the same time, rice and millet were being cultivated in China and Southeast Asia. People moved from villages to cities, to areas of abundant rich grain production near fertile river basins with plenty of water for people, animals, and the irrigation of crops. These cities were the beginnings of the great Agricultural Civilizations. The first Western civilization formed in Mesopotamia where the first cities developed in 4,000 to 3,500 BC. The Tigris and Euphrates Rivers supplied Mesopotamia, or the land between the rivers, just as the Nile River supplied the ancient Egyptian civilization developing during the same time period. Ancient agriculture and civilization spread to Rome, Greece, and Europe, and became the progenitor for European farming and culture.

Yet life in the agricultural societies was far from free of the pressures for survival. Wars were constant in the battle for lands, food, and wealth. Ancient rulers took large shares of food and grain for taxes to use for trade and warfare. The conquered were conscripted into armies and slavery. Floods and drought destroyed crops and livestock, causing famine and starvation for those less powerful without stores of food.

During the agricultural civilizations, the stress to the body was to survive danger and keep a share of the food available. Physical activity was not as intense as that in constant hunting and gathering and the climate was warmer. However, threats to food supply still demanded the need for the shift in metabolism, one that could store food efficiently as fat to survive life-threatening wars and famine by metabolizing more slowly when food was reduced. Cultured grain was the primary means for it to do so. Grain could also be stored to maintain daily supplies between harvests as well as during shorter growing seasons in the colder winter climates to the north.

It is said that the history of grain and bread is the history of civilization. This history is why our bodies crave adequate supplies of bread and its life sustenance. But while bread was important to the early civilizations, there were also many other foods grown in the warm climates that were necessary to nutrition. The many ages of our bodies are dependent on all the earth's natural and wholesome foods. Our bodies are adapted to these foods and metabolize them efficiently for nourishment. They include the carbohydrates in fruits, vegetables, and grains as well as fat and protein. The body needs *all* of these nutrients. Therefore, a diet harmonious to its food history is essential to the body's comfort during weight loss.

We can see how the biological body is accustomed to the food it has depended on to survive throughout genetic history. Each period of time carries with it the effects of the time before and our nutritional needs are cumulative throughout history. This is the food the human body has utilized for many thousands of years and includes hunting and gathering as well as agriculture. We can also see how the body reacts to stress and danger at a biological level to survive. These two factors, the natural need for a balance of foods needed for healthy metabolism and the natural need for less stress and more security to the body are an absolute necessity for successful dieting. Both outright hunger and the hidden hunger must be avoided. *The body must feel it is safe to let go of excessive fat.* To ignore these two factors is to fail to maintain weight loss. Dieting to lose excess fat must be comfortable, secure, and enjoyable. The next chapter reveals more strategy.

8 MAXIMUM CALORIES
SSSA + X(NC + HP + **NH** + MC) = Fat Loss

The key is in giving the body the security of having enough nutritious food o it can relax its need to store fat. Satisfy the body nutritionally and take out the anti-metabolic processed additives of factory-created foods - and it releases fat. This is accomplished by eating the foods it has learned to metabolize in past eras, the foods as close to natural form as possible, rather than those concocted with excess starch, sugar, fat, salt, preservatives, chemical leavenings, and colorings. The ancient natural foods are the real foods the body knows how to metabolize for nourishment and energy. But how many calories are needed?

Not too much and not too little. This is the *Goldilocks Paradigm* (pronounced *pair' a dime*), a pattern or model of thought, used by physicists in the study of the universe. The idea is that basically, everything is balanced and in harmony, as, for example, the stronger and weaker forces in gravity. Not too much and not too little keeps everything "just right." Extremes are not the essence, are not the *raison d'être*, the reason for being. The real essence is somewhere in-between. Take note.

Call to mind Goldilocks, in the Three Bears' house, checks the chairs, beds, and bowls of porridge belonging to Papa Bear, Mama Bear and Baby Bear. She finds Papa and Mama Bear's too much and too little, but Baby Bear's, *for her,* are just right! Not too much and not too little but just right is a model for the universe. It is also a model to use for your diet. This may seem easier said than done. But not with the right game strategy.

The Goldilocks Paradigm for Calorie Counting
Not too much and not too little, but just right. This is the amount of food you can eat and still lose weight without hunger. This is the amount of food you are currently eating. Therefore, to count calories on this diet, you first calculate how many calories you are eating now and set this as your daily upper limit in calories. Some days you will be more hungry and go over the

target amount. Other days, you will eat less. As you lose weight, your target number for calories also declines. *The effect is that the body naturally relaxes its storage of fat as you replace the bad foods with the good foods, because it is now able to metabolize the balanced nutritious food it is given without threats of hunger and insecurity.* Real fat is dissolved too. This is not water weight.

If you are serious about losing excess weight, the question is not whether you need to count calories. The question is how can you not count calories and succeed in the long run. If you don't count calories, you are using someone else's lopsided starvation diet. Calorie counting is the only sane way to mathematically and scientifically keep track of what you are eating with freedom, choice, and nutrition. Meanwhile you learn the calorie values of different foods and learn how to read food labels, so necessary to industrial food life. However, diets that restrict calories to severe limits are not the answer either. We've discussed previously how and why nutritionally unbalanced and severely restricted diets end up being counterproductive and even dangerous to health as correctly perceived by the body with hunger and cravings.

How many calories are you now eating to support you current weight? To calculate this amount, simply multiply your current weight by 12 (an energy factor explained later):

Calculating Total Calories with Energy Factor

Your current weight_____x 12 = _____Your total daily calories.

For example, if you weigh 185 pounds, that amount will be 185 x 12 = 2220 calories, your upper calorie limit for the day. As you eat your own target calories of the good foods in the menu, your body automatically reduces fat, without hunger! As you lose weight, say every five to ten pounds, you will reduce your upper limit in calories. In the above example, after weight reduces to 180 pounds, the upper calorie limit is 2160, at 175 pounds, the upper range is 2100. The beauty of this diet is that you will lose weight while eating within 10 pounds or more of your upper range in calories, if you are eating the metabolism-tuning food (it does not include the processed starch and sugar foods). In the above example, weighing 185, this would be anywhere from 2280 calories to 2160 calories. One reason for this is that calories in foods differ as to how much of the food is actually converted to metabolic energy rather than to fat stores. And natural foods, the X Factor foods, are metabolized more efficiently with some of the nutrients feeding the processes of metabolism. Of course, individuals vary and you will be able to experiment as to how many calories you can eat and still lose weight without hunger.

By putting calories per pound with the 12 factor to work for yourself, you can compare each day's calorie intake and weight to see how calories and weight interact. *You can also see how your body, on its own, without processed overly refined starch and sugar, is asking (with hunger, which you immediately satisfy with the good foods) for calories just under those required to maintain overweight, with the effect of reducing fat.* To repeat, as you eat to prevent hunger, but without processed starch and sugar products, you will see how your body, *on its own*, decreases calorie demand. You immediately feel better and have more energy. That sluggish, sleepy, dragged out, drugged up feeling goes away. The feeling of well being is so great, you will gladly continue your diet. After all, you are not starving, you are not hungry, and you are replacing empty fat producing calories with the nutritious food your body so desperately appreciates. The body, rather than being signaled to store fat for famine, now feels comfortable with the abundance of nutritious more easily metabolized food, dairy products, meat, fruits, and vegetables. The body adapts for the "good times" of abundant food supply, close to the land, with good weather and water.

You'll also feel less stress and have more energy and time for activity you enjoy. Excessive eating of processed starch and sugar dampens the body fires and produces feelings of tiredness and depression. You will be truly amazed with the difference.

Your Daily Weight and Calorie Journal

As you begin to diet with a new understanding of how foods familiar to the body through the ages are more easily and "cleanly" metabolized, without residues stored as fat, then eating these kinds of foods should reduce fat, regardless of the number of calories. This does happen with this diet, once excessively manufactured foods, refined starch and refined sugar, are replaced with the good familiar foods of earth and time. Yet, as already mentioned, the dieter needs more direction and guidance than just foregoing certain foods in order to stay focused on the diet. The temptation of perceived satisfaction is everywhere in the food environment. It's just too easy to stray once, twice, and thrice, then back to the old eating habits. This is why a *Daily Weight and Calorie Journal* is needed. You are able to see for yourself immediate effects of certain foods (such as fast food). This will prove to you that real foods are not fattening. You can see on paper the record of what you have eaten and what you weigh each day. You need to weigh yourself each morning before eating or drinking, without clothes or in the same type clothes each day. You will then list the foods you eat that day and total the calories. You can also write down as many or as few of your thoughts of the day as you wish, your feelings and actions, what is occurring in your life. You are then more aware of stress and frustration and their possible influences on your eating habits. When you feel good, you can also make note. Your *Daily Weight and Calorie Journal* is a personal part of the adventure into yourself as you lose weight. Any piece of paper and pencil will do as will any format you choose, but keep each day's record so you can refer back to it and see progress. A sample is included at the end of the chapter.

Calories as Life Energy

The *minimum* number of calories needed by the body is around 1,000 to 1,200 a day. This is why reducing diets usually begin with these limits. Basic bodily functions are still nourished while fat stores are burned. (However, you are *really* hungry, a situation you want to avoid. Read on for the solution.) If fewer than 1,000 calories a day are consumed, the body slows down, metabolic rates decrease, and weight reduction slows. The body braces "to survive the famine." When calories are inadequate for the body's needs and there are no fat stores, starvation develops as the body cannot maintain and repair itself. Body organs fail and muscles shrink to produce the energy to survive. In ancient times, this meant the last possibility for survival. Glamorous models and movie stars on starvation diets have suffered permanent heart and organ damage. Anorexics and bulimics, alternately gorging with food, then purging to the point of starvation, can die from damage to their organs as they starve themselves to death. Medicine is indicating, rightly so, that the eating disorders originate, not only as psychiatric problems, but in malnutrition or in lack of the adequate nutrition from the variety of foods needed by the body. The body is thrown into chaos and desperation, trying to get the food it needs. And how often do these famous stars turn to drugs in place of eating to achieve those skinny contours, only to end up in rehab or worse.

Overweight itself needs extra calories to maintain its fat. More energy is required to support and move around the extra weight all day. The heart, lungs, muscles, the entire body, work harder, consuming more calories and energy, fighting through the extra fat to function. A fatter body has more skin to maintain and more blood circulation routes to supply the fat. It takes more energy to carry around that extra fat, whether it's ten pounds or 40 pounds. The more fat, the more weight, the more energy needed to maintain it.

Calories are "burned" or expended even while at rest. Sleeping uses around 50 calories an hour or 350 calories for seven hours. (Again, the number depends on body size.) Sitting and watching television uses about 60 calories an hour; eating while doing so expends about 80 calories an hour. More activity such as playing golf uses as many as 300 calories an hour.

The body adapts to what's done to it as best it can. For example, if alcohol is consumed regularly *in place of food*, the body learns to look to alcohol for calories, resulting in alcoholism. If the body gets cheeseburgers for nourishment, it wants cheeseburgers. If the body has received extra calories and is storing and maintaining fat, it wants to continue to do so. The body is programmed to adapt for survival in the environment. The body adapts in order to survive, to maintain homeostasis and harmony. When the body feels nervous, stressed, threatened, it wants to do something about it. Getting extra food and storing it as fat is a way to protect itself from the perceived insecurities, for the famine ahead.

All foods are not equal and therefore not all calories are equal. Some clog metabolism and create fat. This means that manufactured foods altered from their natural state are extremely alien to the body and are more readily stored as fat as the body tries to deal with them. The body needs *natural* carbohydrates such as fruits and whole grains and has tolerance for *natural* yeast breads, pasta, unleavened breads, and whole grains in about the same proportion during the week as the history of humankind without, then with, bread and flour during agriculture. This is why these foods are part of the weekly "sometimes" foods in the losing-weight diet menu. You will learn you do not have to give up delicious breads and pastas. *After* stopping the addiction to processed starch and sugar, *after* eating the increased protein and the fruits and vegetables and dairy products for a few days, you should satisfy the urge for natural bread and pasta type food and enjoy it fully. This is described in previous chapters. The object of this diet is to make you and your body happy and secure, not tortured and deprived. However, you do need to continue to count the calories while losing weight. During and after weight loss, you will find your enjoyment of these type foods within reason will not result in weight gain. And after losing the desired weight, you will not need to count calories and will be able to *easily* maintain your weight.

12 Factor

Why multiply weight by 12 to figure calories? This figure represents the number of calories or energy per pound used by a sedentary to moderately active person. This number was determined from an average in tables giving the spread of calories needed each day based on height. As an average, it reflects the relatively inactive lifestyle most of us live in walking to the car or bus, walking around the supermarket, sitting at a desk, watching TV, or working at a computer.

Calorie rate per pound is similar to the miles per gallon your vehicle gets out of the gasoline it burns and which varies according to vehicle type, driving conditions, speed, weight, acceleration, etc., but is an *average* of miles per gallon used. In much the same way, you can figure how many average calories your body is using per pound of body weight.

The factor would be larger for those moderately active, say 15 (doing yard work or housework), and larger still for heavy labor such as construction, at 16, 17, and more. Children also have higher energy factors because they are still growing. These calculations are based on the National Academy of Sciences recommended daily calories for average weights and are amounts for maintaining weight, not losing weight. You can see these amounts vary so that determining a common useful figure for everyone is challenging. This is why the factor is flexible. Only experience can show you the best amount that works for you to lose weight without hunger. If you are hungry and are going over your daily calories, experiment with a higher number, starting at 15. The correct average number is the one that allows you to steadily lose weight without hunger. However the 12 factor is a good average. Using this factor allows you to lose weight eating around this range of calories. And multiplying it times weight already figures in size and energy differences for bigger people who expend more energy supporting more weight. The key is eating the metabolizer foods in place of the foods that stifle metabolism.

You can also use the 12 factor to figure how much "weight you ate that day," i.e. how much you would weigh if you ate that many calories every day. For example, if you ate 2000 calories during the day, at an energy level of 12 calories per pound, the weight rate you ate would be 2000 divided by 12 = 166 pounds.

Therefore, eating an average of 2000 calories every day with a sedentary lifestyle would likely result in a weight around 166 pounds.

What is your target weight? You can also multiply that by 12 to figure how many calories per day would result in that weight. For example, you want to reduce to 140 pounds and activity level is around 12 calories per pound: 140 x 12 = 1680 calories per day. However, to avoid hunger you will find you want to eat the calories around your current weight, not your target weight. Calorie needs will decrease as your weight decreases.

As an option, you can also figure your actual energy factor your body is using as you lose weight on the diet by totaling all your daily weights and all the calories and dividing to find the calorie rate per pound your body is using to lose weight. Example: (/ is divided by)

Tracking Metabolic Rate			
Day	Weight	Calories	Calorie Rate Per Pound
Day 1	200	2400	2400/200 = 12
Day 2	200	2395	2395/200 = 11.98
Day 3	197	2495	2495/197 = 12.66
Day 4	196	2250	2250/196 = 11.48
Day 5	195	2195	2195/195 = 11.26
Totals	988	11735	11735/988 = 11.88

This sample resulted in an average calorie rate of 11.88 calories per pound while losing weight, without hunger, on the diet. This is real fat loss and not water weight. This figure is based on gradually decreasing weight and for our purposes here, represents the metabolic rate the body is using to decrease fat stores. Each day's calories will yield a different amount in the ebb and flow, rising and falling, living and breathing, natural metabolism. This is why, on a daily basis, it is best to use a fixed rate of 12. This gives a consistent figure for comparison. However, if you calculate your energy rate at a much different level and it is working to control hunger while losing excess fat, you can use your own number.

To begin however, you need only figure your upper range for calories by multiplying your weight times 12. You will probably see that the result is close to the same number of calories your body currently wants without strong urges to eat more. If the 12 factor seems too low and you want more calories, as mentioned, raise the level to 15 or more. As long as your hunger is controlled and *excess fat is melting away*, proven by your daily morning weigh-in, the factor is flexible and open to experimentation.

The energy factor is an estimated if not theoretical figure. Its importance is in helping you to visualize your weight loss and weight goal in metabolic terms. It translates calories into weight. This helps you lose weight gradually without going hungry. It helps you see how the body is adjusting to the diet by gradually and naturally decreasing the number of calories it needs while decreasing unhealthy fat stores. Otherwise you may fail to see how effectively the diet is working and give up under the false impression that if you are not suffering, you are not losing weight.

While numbers are only average indicators of life processes that are constantly changing they are very helpful for providing a basis for direction and comparison. With your numbers before you, you can see your progress and remain confident. This is especially helpful when your body resists going below certain weight levels and plateaus there. An initial reduction in weight is not felt as threatening to body harmony. However, after a few days, the body will poise to maintain the current weight and want a few more calories. Go with it with healthy food and remain steady on the diet. You will find your body will gradually adjust and gently agree to drop a few more pounds. These plateaus can be especially stubborn but don't push it too much. Give in to hunger and eat a little more of the good food. The amount will still be close to your 12 factor calculation. As you lose weight, without hunger and struggle, the calorie demand will slowly decrease and you will be satisfied with less food. (A smaller vehicle uses less gas; a lighter body uses fewer calories.) *Calorie counting really helps here, so you don't feel that you are just "groping in the dark" or that the diet is not working.* Also, this applies only if you are eating the good foods. A plateau here means staying at the same weight, not gaining weight. A gain surely means you have eaten the LTN foods.

Ideals in Body Weight

The next matter at hand is how much do you weigh? Are you overweight? How much do you need to lose to feel comfortable?

There is some question as to what the ideal body weight should be. Whether being ten pounds underweight, that is, being under the amounts on the charts for average weights, is healthier or not, is still being researched. After all, it takes lifetime studies to determine whether being slightly underweight promotes health and longevity. Of course, skinny looks good on camera and as a clothes hanger for high fashion clothing. But is it healthy? Your own aesthetic should be what feels best to you. If you find skinny scary, it probably is, to your body. The average height and weight charts relied on so much in the past have fallen out of favor. The weights were much too low. It was found that longevity in older people seemed to follow a trend with being slightly overweight, around ten pounds, but not obese. This has led to much more relaxed ranges for healthy weights, such as in the BMI calculations found online. BMI helps figure the amounts or percentages of body fat considered healthy and the amounts not healthy.

Charts and tables indicate only areas of healthy weight and overweight. You owe it to yourself to find the weight that feels best to you. You may have a weight in mind that felt great in the past, perhaps before belly fat. For most people, as they lose weight, the belly fat is last to go. The legs, thighs, arms, chest lose fat before that around the middle. From the body's point of view, this makes sense. The fat most immediately accessible, protecting organs against the cold and famine, is closest to the digestive organs and the body central. Usually, belly fat (hip fat for some) is the last to go. You may want to plan to reduce to a point ridding yourself of excess belly fat. Again this is a matter for individuals. After you've lost the really oppressive fat, you may decide a little cushion around the belly feels best to you.

Of course, exercise can help with more uniform and proportionate weight loss over the entire body. It also burns more calories. The conflict the body feels with reduced calories and heavy exercise is understandable. What does it mean biologically? That it's time to utilize fat stores for the crisis, the famine, the hunt. Go get food! Hunt. Gather. Move. As stated before, these are reasons why successful weight reduction should be gradual and stress free, without hunger and over-exertion.

Gradual steady weight loss and light exercise will allow your body time to adapt without signaling that more food is needed. As you choose your way through this diet, you will see the pounds melt away. Counting calories and weighing yourself will help you see the process mathematically. Not too much and not too little. And just right for you.

A World of Calories Simplified

The world of calories can be a complicated one. Calorie counts for foods are often listed in strange amounts such as 3.5 ounces. This is because the scientific measurements were done for 100 grams. One gram is around .035 ounces, so 100 grams equals a little over 3.5 ounces. This makes it difficult to figure the different amounts you are eating, such as 4 ounces. This is why *Love Your Diet Calorie Counter*, available separately, gives calories for a small measure, such as one ounce, in Measure A, which can then simply be multiplied by the number of ounces eaten. Measure B gives an amount for an average serving. Calorie amounts are also rounded to the nearest 5 where reasonable to make calculation easier. The calorie amounts for LTN Foods however are not rounded. This is also explained in the calorie counter. Most packaged foods, such as sour cream, yogurt, and milk already have calories listed on the container. However, fresh produce and bakery products do not have calories listed. Nor do fast foods and restaurant foods provide calories as a rule, although this is changing somewhat. This makes calorie counting a potentially gymnastic chore and is a primary reason why dieters prefer not to have to count calories. If you stray from the diet, keep counting calories and weighing yourself! The diet is forgiving and you will not immediately gain weight by giving in to temptation or circumstance. However, if you overdo it, you will see dramatic proof in your daily weigh-in that your body cannot easily metabolize highly processed and fast fat foods. Your daily morning weigh-in is your proof of what foods are easily metabolized and those that are not.

You also need to maintain your protein intake levels to a number at around 1/2 your targeted body weight. For example, if you should weigh 160 pounds, your protein should equal as much as 80 grams, more or less, for the day. Maintaining protein levels also helps control hunger. In the *Calorie Counter*, available separately, protein levels are given for Measure B, an average serving. EAAs or complete proteins are highlighted or asterisked. (Due to space and formatting limitations, protein amounts are only listed in the printed edition.) While nearly all foods contain protein, for the diet, count only these major sources of protein such as meat and dairy or nutrition drinks to maintain your levels to at least 15 to 20 grams intake for breakfast, 20 to 30 grams intake during the day, and 20 to 30 grams for dinner. As discussed earlier, major protein foods contain complete proteins needed by the body. Other foods contain lesser amounts or incomplete proteins and their protein levels are also listed in the charts as a matter of interest and to indicate protein sources that supplement the major protein players.

You will need the following items to keep track of your weight and calories.

Weighing, Measuring, Counting Supplies

Weight scale -- for weighing yourself each morning before eating or drinking.

Food scale -- for weighing food in serving sizes in ounces up to at least a pound

Individual measuring cups – 2 C, 1 C, ½ C, ¼ C   (C= Cup)

1 Tablespoon measure – T (tablespoon in the diet)

1 teaspoon measure – tsp (teaspoon in the diet)

Calculator – optional but advised

***Love Your Diet Calorie Counter* –** foods to eat, not to eat, and their calories

Your Daily Weight and Calorie Journal – sample format at end of chapter

9 DIET GUIDE
SSSA + X(NC + HP + NH + MC) = Fat Loss

In the previous chapters, we've explained and discussed each aspect of the diet including the necessity to *Stop Starch and Sugar Addiction* and what the *X Factor* has to do with food choices and metabolism. We discussed how you need to eat all kinds of *Natural Carbohydrates* and *High Protein* foods in dairy and meats for healthy, comfortable weight loss. We emphasized the importance of *No Hunger* and how to plan *Maximum Calories* with the Goldilocks Paradigm.

We learned how and why nutrition is essential to healthy weight and a healthy body. We presented a loving, caring, natural eating strategy to lose excess fat and maintain weight by replacing the torture and ineffectiveness of traditional and fad diets. In the next chapter are some basic menus and lists of food choices to get started. But first, let's summarize diet basics and then look at some helpful tips in putting the plan to work. Some of the material has been stated before, but reminders are helpful.

Body and Mind
Your instincts for nutritious food will be awakened once you give up the foods that have been stifling your metabolism and stacking on the pounds. The tremendous release your body feels in SSSA, Stopping Starch & Sugar Addiction to processed foods with the accompanying additives of excess sugar, salt, fat, starch, and chemicals feels so good it is as though your body is saying *thank you!*

You'll gladly head for the produce section at the market for natural carbohydrates and natural sugars. You'll want to eat voluptuous fruit and rich lush vegetables. Over the weeks, your body will direct you to green and leafy, golden and fruity, to living colors in shades of yellow, red, purple, and orange, as you experience metabolic release.

In the beginning, *off factory-created and processed starch and sugar,*

51

you'll want to indulge in the foods your body has been missing, foods with natural nutrients, foods your body already knows it needs to metabolize excess fats. Choose the ones your body *wants* to eat, the ones which seem to reach out and extend an invitation to bite into them and absorb their sustenance.

At the market, look at all the fruits and vegetables. Which ones do you *want* to eat? Reach out and pick them up. Smell the fruit. Is it ripe? Sweet? Ask the store produce manager for a sample if unsure. Juicy sweet fruit is important for this indulgence and it needs to deliver the taste it promises.

Take it all with you and eat all you want of these fresh fruits and vegetables. You may be amazed at how much of it you want to eat, especially if you have picked it out with care and it is good produce. Your body seems to be starved for this food.

Fully indulge your inclinations to feast on fruits and vegetables. You are replacing the addictive starch and sugar with natural sugars and nutrients. Let your body know that times are good. Food is abundant. No famine ahead. Yet your mind must also play a role with action follows thought, planning and reflection, logic and reason. By weighing yourself and counting calories, the mind is a believer too. The body is seen increasingly as an instrument of the mind. Yet the body, the human, the organism, is a fully functioning sum of the parts. We suffer when we neglect the body's most basic needs for feelings of harmony in its environment with good food and nutrition, adequate sleep, and freedom from stress.

The body has its own requirements in metabolizing food for life energy although it is amazingly adaptable, always working hard to repair and renew, using the food, water, and air available to it. We know the body needs nutrients in this process, such as protein, carbohydrates, fats, vitamins and minerals. The body gives messages, in the form of a want, a need, an attention, to foods that will best produce needed nutrients for metabolic processes, once the excessive processed starch and sugar is given up. If the body is storing excess fat, this is a symptom of something wrong.

When the body is storing and then stressfully struggling with excess starch and sugar, with strange chemicals and additives, it is working hard to manage what it is given in order to survive. But metabolism is dampened and the body needs more. It wants to keep eating, to find the nutrients from past adaptations. This creates feelings of addiction to food as the body attempts to regulate its own processes without needed nutrients. This lack is felt in the body as a stress in the environment to which preparation for survival must occur. And fat is stored for the tough times ahead, for the famine. Yet the body works and yearns for the time of harmony, when adequate nutrition signals rest and optimum metabolism. Excessive refined starch and sugar smothers and confuses these metabolic adjustments by the body. By giving them up and recognizing the forces of addiction, your body is then free to signal its true needs. But you must pay attention, listen, and be in touch with your own body. Give it a chance to indicate what it needs without the SSA. You will be surprised to learn that it really doesn't want the foods you have been eating when it has the real nutrition. This diet is an adventure into yourself.

Do eat as much as your body wants *without* refined carbohydrates and refined sugar. You will see the amount is around your current weight. The idea is to reduce gradually, not all at once, so you are feeding the body, not torturing it with denial. Again, some days you'll want more calories, some days less. This is another reason weighing yourself and counting calories is important. You'll see the adjustments the body is making rather than giving up a diet because you feel it is failing. The weight loss is sure and steady but you need to see it in writing to get the total picture.

If you feel you want some candy, then have some. But do not eat it in place of the nutritious food. Assure yourself it's still there if needed. Have a piece. As you eat more natural sugars, such as those in fruit, you'll find you don't want many sugared products. The whole impetus of this diet is that you eat what you choose to eat within the guidelines of LTN, Little-to-No highly processed products along with adequate protein intake, fresh fruits and vegetables, and natural whole grains.

You have to experience this diet to truly understand how wonderful you will feel. You will want to indulge at first in all the wonderful nutrients your body has been missing, such as eating *many* helpings of fruit, but this will level out. You will feel like you are feasting on a gourmet diet and so you are. And your slimming shape will make you feel light and alive. SSSA, Stop Starch and Sugar Addiction. Get plenty of protein. Then let your body help guide you to the good foods it not only needs but wants. *(This only happens if you truly give up the refined starch and sugar foods).*

As you continue to feast on real foods, the ancient, the natural foods your body needs, yet continue to lose pounds, you'll be amazed at how much you can eat of all the good foods, still lose weight, and then easily maintain weight. Others, when they see what you are eating and weighing, will think you are starving yourself behind the scenes, when in fact you aren't going even a little bit hungry! You've only been enjoying the best of foods such as rich buttery avocadoes, crisp cucumbers, and big fluffy baked potatoes dripping in sour cream.

Universal – Fish Cakes & Lobster
This is a universal diet, which can be followed regardless of culture or income because it reverts to ancient natural foods that are timeless. Money spent on the more expensive manufactured foods, such as canned soups and frozen dinners, can be directed to fresh fruits and vegetables. Potatoes are less expensive than potato chips. Yogurt is a reasonable expense,

especially in place of meat protein. Beans along with meat provide complete protein. Many soy products such as tofu are inexpensive. Canned fish is inexpensive. Canned salmon and mackerel make good fishcakes. In other words, you don't have to spend a fortune on this diet. This diet is for everyone who can adapt it to every socioeconomic scale and every culture.

Depending on where you live, such as in a cold climate in a smaller town, fruit can be one of the more expensive items on the menu. But you have to figure in what you are giving up instead in manufactured sugar and starch. That boxed sugary cereal, those cookies on the shelf, empty cakes, shelf bread so limp, lifeless, and full of air, it doesn't satisfy anything, these foods are not inexpensive. Compare the price per pound for your favorite empty snack food with the price per pound for fresh nutritious fruit. The point is that our values are distorted when it comes to the convenience foods marketed to us. Note that sugary sweets are outrageously priced, due to supply and demand. In other words, in place of empty starch and sugar, you can afford to feast on fresh vegetables, rice, champagne and caviar, and lobster you cook yourself.

Choose X Factor Ancient Real Foods

These foods are not fattening because they can be metabolized efficiently. This includes all the natural carbohydrates. When is a food an ancient link, a metabolic food? Ask yourself if it has been eaten as a significant part of human history, in the Stone Age and in the Agricultural Age before Industrial Age manufacturing. The body still needs its nutrients in as natural a form as possible. Eating this food is very satisfying and gratifying. Fish, fruits, vegetables, grains are examples of foods our bodies still need whether we were raised eating them or not or whether we choose to eat them or not. Cupcakes on the shelf are not an ancient food. A peach, a date, a pistachio nut, these are ancient foods. Milk, bread, olive oil, and wine are ancient foods. Natural sugar cane, not refined white sugar, is an ancient food.

Avoid Manufactured Foods

These are foods new to the body in alien forms created by manufacturing in the past 200 years with the Industrial Revolution. The body does not have the coding to efficiently deal with them. Food products made with highly refined sugar and flour throw the metabolism out of balance and create feelings of addiction. With many other convenience foods such as frozen dinners, the body gets less protein, more starch fillers, less nutrition, and more calories than when eating the more natural foods it needs.

Complete lists of the menu foods or what to eat and LTN Foods or what not to eat are in the next chapter. The *Love Your Diet Calorie Counters* are also conveniently separated into what to eat and not to eat. However, choosing the right foods is easy. The choice of food to eat is the unaltered natural, the link food, people have eaten through the ages. The food not to eat is manufactured, highly processed, highly sugared food. Note the following choices. Which foods are not fattening?

Choosing Natural Foods

1		2
apple	vs	apple-flavored toaster pastry
peanuts	vs	peanut butter cookies
baked potato	vs	potato chips
popcorn or fresh corn	vs	corn chips
natural whole grain cereal	vs	boxed cereal that has been formed into shapes
honey	vs	refined white sugar
70% cacao chocolate bar	vs	regular candy bar

The first choices in column 1 are the natural non-fattening ancient or real foods, those to eat.

We're not promoting extremes in that *no* artificial or manufactured anything should ever be eaten. This is a real world diet taking advantage of all food choices to lose weight naturally, nutritiously, and without hunger. Artificial sweeteners are a good example. They are especially helpful in not feeling deprived when first quitting heavily sugared products but you should not continue them or use them regularly. No sugar added ice cream is another example. Of course children should not have artificial sweeteners with unknown effect on growing bodies. They should eat the all natural ice cream.

Lowfat Dairy Products

Include an ample supply as indicated in the menu guide. Take them to work with you along with fruit to prevent hunger. The milk sugars also help stop starch and sugar addiction. Dairy foods are rich in nutrients: carbohydrates, protein, fats, vitamins, and minerals. Yogurt is rich in B-complex vitamins. Cottage cheese is high in protein. The dairy products are a very important part of the diet as satisfying, less expensive protein choices that help you to be calm, peaceful, even tranquil, on this diet. However, manufactured cheese is recommended as a go-easy food as it may be constipating and slow down digestion due to additives in processing. However, natural cheeses should be fine. For the yogurt in the diet, as mentioned, mix two tablespoons or more of the lowfat artificially sweetened yogurt with all natural yogurts for both taste and nutrition, the LYD yogurt.

Meat, Fish, and Poultry.

Plan at least one major meal of the day with meat protein, whether beef, pork, fish, or poultry. Fish, shellfish, and fowl are somewhat lower in calories and seem to be more easily metabolized than beef or pork, probably due to the fact that fish and poultry are more ancient foods as people lived near coasts and waterways with fish, water birds and eggs. Frozen fish products, such as the fillets with batter-coatings are an exception to trying not to use convenience food on this diet because they are consistent, easy, and have good protein. They are extremely handy and easy to use after a day at work and contribute to continued weight loss. Just place in a skillet and heat. The oil is in the batter. Fresh fish is of course better, if truly fresh. If it smells very fishy, it is not fresh. Fish that is not fresh is the biggest difficulty to eating much of it. However, frozen fillets that are flash-frozen are more predictable.

Preserved meats such as hot dogs, sausage, and lunchmeat are not recommended as good choices because of the preservatives, additives, salt, and high saturated fat content. However, if you want these products, you can experiment to see if they work for you in losing weight or whether they cause weight gain. (Weigh yourself the next morning after eating hot dogs or sausage and potato chips. They can stay on the body for 3 to 4 days.) So many choices, but a little knowledge and a game plan makes all the difference.

Soy Products

You may not be a tofu fan but it's worth a try. Soybeans are rich in protein and tofu is made from soybean curd. Just three ounces of tofu has 7 grams of complete protein. Firm tofu sliced and cooked in a pan of oil until lightly brown tastes like fluffy egg whites. Or it can be used uncooked. Tofu is nearly tasteless on its own, readily taking up the flavor of other liquids or seasonings, such as soy sauce. It can be added to rice, vegetables, soups, and sauces for added protein. There are many interesting recipes for tofu and miso, another soy product, on the internet, which are worth checking out and will help make you a believer if not one already.

Veggie burgers or meatless patties are made of soybeans and are tasty. They can be found in the frozen food case. Mixes are also available in bulk foods in supermarkets or in organic food stores. Just mix with water and fry in oil.

Nutrition drinks high in protein are often made of soybeans and are excellent protein supplements. There is a question as to whether *concentrated* soy products stimulate hormone based breast cancer. If this is a question for you, stay with whey based protein drinks. Tofu is natural and not concentrated.

Fruit

Fresh raw fruit is very convenient to eat. Simply wash, then pare and slice as needed. The challenge of fruit is in the shopping where you need to pick out the best. Smell is a good indicator as to how ripe it is and how it will taste. However, some of the fruit in the supermarket is kept cool and has little smell. When uncertain as to quality, purchase only a little and if satisfactory, go back and get more. Produce workers will usually give you a sample taste of the fruit if you ask them if it is sweet and ripe. Nothing is more discouraging when eating fruit than unripe, sour fruit. This is why some give up trying different fruits and stick to bananas. And while bananas are a wonderful food, you need a variety of juicy fruits of many choices and colors for more nutrition and better metabolism.

There are many elaborate schemes to protect fruit to market, some producing fruit that spoils before it is ever ripe! It doesn't have to be that way. Consumers can make a difference. Be picky. You can also return fruit to the store if it in unacceptable. Keep your receipts until you are satisfied. Don't give up. Once you have gained the knack for picking out and obtaining good fruit, you will be very happy. If you are dieting during the summer or in warm climates during growing seasons, fruit is more plentiful and offers more choices. Go to the local farmer's market where you will be surrounded by deliciously ripe invitations.

You will also find that you probably do not want fruit juice when eating the whole fruit. The whole fruit supplies bulk and sustenance that fruit juice does not. Also sample the seeds and eat as much skin as is palatable. Thoroughly wash all your fruit. As an added note, some prefer good fruit at room temperature, as it seems to enhance flavor and to be more pleasant on the palate. The thorough enjoyment of fruit is crucial to your dieting enjoyment and success.

Prepare Vegetables

In the past, you may have thought nothing of baking up a batch of manufactured refrigerator dough cookies while preparing vegetables seemed a big chore. This will change on this diet as you give up refined starch and sugar addiction. Raw fresh vegetables you prepare yourself won't have additives such as coloring, salt, and preservatives. Cutting up a cucumber, slicing a tomato, or cooking some brussels sprouts take little time and effort. On this diet, you will feel so good you will look forward to preparing these foods to eat.

Cooking adds to the variety and amounts of vegetables on your menu. You can steam vegetables over water on top of the range. Just place them in a pan with a lid. A rack that holds them up out of the water is good for retaining nutrients and keeping them from getting waterlogged. Or, you can sauté vegetables in good vegetable oil. (You can make your own wilted spinach by simply placing fresh spinach over other food as it cooks.)

As for the microwave, experiment as to what tastes the best to you when cooking raw vegetables. In some cases it makes little difference while in others the food is dry, tough, and tasteless. Frozen vegetables also may be an additional time saver and retain nutrients, but they also may not be as satisfying as fresh cooked.

Vegetables are packed with essential vitamins and minerals and have very few calories. They are *big metabolism tuners!* Plan *large* servings of plump hot vegetables for serious eating with lowfat sour cream or butter.

Salads

Green salads have been so much a part of dieting that observation alone could prove that salads cause weight gain. Of course salads are good for everyone. But they do not provide much bulk. A bowl of lettuce isn't much food, so green salad alone cannot fulfill the increased need for the nutrition of a world of vegetables in the diet. Salad dressing is also usually heaped up and overused. Lettuce for green salad can also be time consuming to prepare and store. You do not have to make salad all the time out of feelings of diet duty or have the traditional green salad at all. You can easily forego salad and just wash and slice up the raw salad vegetables by themselves. You can then pick through a truly full plate of radishes, cucumbers, tomatoes, carrots, or any other raw vegetables you like.

Desserts

Desserts polish off a meal and make it feel more complete, especially after dinner. Desserts are a pleasure made with ripe, sweet, juicy fruits. Natural enhancers, such as honey and cream or whipped cream can be added. The artificial whipped topping on fruit or on artificially sweetened gelatin or pudding adds a touch of luxury, especially when first giving up refined sugars. Artificially sweetened ice cream (no refined sugar added) is delicious in a banana split (or with any fruit) with peanuts, 1 to 2 tablespoons chocolate sauce, and whipped topping. However, most ice cream tastes best if some natural fat is left in. The nonfat, nonsugar kind can be very tasteless though personal preference varies. Some of the nonsugar fruit pies are also very good and can fill in as a sometimes food with ice cream or whipped topping. However, artificial sweeteners should be regarded *only as a temporary solution* as you switch to the natural sugars and lose your addiction to refined white sugar.

Fats and Oils

A good olive oil is tasty and heavy enough to fry meats and sauté vegetables without sticking. Olive oil and garlic cloves make any meal a feast. Purchase a huge container so you will use it liberally. Olive oil is monounsaturated rather than polyunsaturated and a nutritional favorite. Choose cold pressed, first press olive oil for fresh nutrition.

The polyunsaturated (liquid at room temperature) vegetable oils are also good, but it is recommended that you watch omega 6 and omega 3 balance. Most vegetable oils are omega 6 but can be balanced out with the omega 3 in coldwater fish oil, flaxseed oil, and canola oil. Soybean oil also has some omega 3.

Some low calorie margarines are good and some are quite watery. A product made with butter and yogurt is quite tasty and low in calories. Butter is also back in favor but is high in calories at 100 calories per tablespoon.

There are delicious salad dressings on the market that are very low calorie. You will need to experiment as to which ones taste good to you.
Lowfat everything is good on any diet. Meat should be lean. But the body needs a certain amount of fat. Remember that fats and oils have 100 to 125 calories per tablespoon, which naturally requires restraint.

Eat with Fingers More Often
The biological body needs to feel the security of touching food. People have eaten with their hands for many thousands of years while eating using utensils is fairly recent. Note that a major attraction of many fast foods are that most are eaten using the fingers and hands!

Maintain Balance in Foods
Eat varieties of fruit, vegetables, and protein foods. Remember that our metabolism requires many different nutrients.

Cook More Food on Top of the Range
The range is not the ancient campfire but the effect is similar. We need to be involved with our food and get satisfaction out of seeing it being prepared. We like to smell and see food as it cooks. With the food in the open, we can readily add seasonings and be more creative.

Salt
There's way too much of it in prepared foods for flavor enhancement. The effect is thirst and water retention. Most foods already have natural salt. By using more unprocessed foods, you have more control over the amount of salt being used. Make certain the salt you do use is iodized. This adds the iodine our bodies need based on the inherited need for the iodine in seafood.

Herbs and Spices
Sensations to the taste buds. Experiment using more herbs and spices for

flavor. Unlike salt, they have little bits of all kinds of vitamins and minerals in the small portions used. Paprika, chili powder and cayenne are rich in Vitamin A and contain B vitamins, Vitamin C, iron, phosphorous, calcium, selenium, zinc, and potassium. (1 teaspoon of paprika is very rich in Vitamin A with 1107 IU.) Spices such as cinnamon and herbs such as basil, marjoram, oregano, parsley, and sage contain vitamins and minerals as well as small amounts of plant proteins and fats.

Condiments
They can be used liberally, just watch the calories. Regular mayonnaise has 100 calories per tablespoon because it is a fat made from oil. Lowfat mayo has only 40 calories.. Soy sauce has only 10 calories per tablespoon; seafood and cocktail sauce, only 15-20 calories per tablespoon. The juice of a fresh lemon is a wonderful flavor enhancement. Good condiments complement a meal and should not be avoided for a few little calories. Check the labels.

Clean Out Refrigerator
Get rid of everything that's been there for months and years. Now that you will be eating fresh fruits and vegetables, the contents of your refrigerator will be beautiful with shapes and colors.

Clean Out Cupboards
Throw out all the crackers, cookies, chips, pastries, empty cardboard cereals in colors and shapes, imitation syrups, and sugared punch imitating juice. You will need to replace these snack foods with the nuts, seeds, fruits, etc. listed in the menus.

Use Your Freezer
Buying a large package of chicken breasts or thighs or fresh fish fillets and packaging them in serving sizes in the freezer will provide convenient meals. Just thaw in the microwave and sauté with olive oil and garlic or your favorite seasonings. Or place in marinade in the refrigerator in the morning for preparing that evening. *A successful diet depends on having the foods you are eating available at all times with a minimum of effort.*

Eat a Good Breakfast High in Protein
Breakfast provides a base for the entire day in preventing hunger and having plenty of energy. Plan a breakfast of at least 15 to 20 grams of protein.

Grocery List
Make a list before you go to the store. This will save you money and reduce impulse buying, especially for LTN foods. It will also keep you focused on

your diet plan. However, do leave room on your list for impulse and bargains in the fruit and vegetable department.

The Produce Department
Pause and look. Look at all the selections and "listen" to your body. Pick out what you *want* to eat. Try something new you've never eaten before.

Read the Labels
Prepared foods have labels listing ingredients such as calories, fats, fiber, protein, carbohydrates, sugar, sodium, and some include vitamin and mineral content.

Think About What You Eating and How It Feels Later
For example, some butter substitutes may be low in calories, but taste bad and feel bad afterwards. Warning signs to drop and replace a food are feeling turned off, bloated, thirsty, slow, sluggish.

Water
Drink water before drinking other beverages. That way, you are not interpreting the need for water as the need for another diet soda, cup of coffee, or glass of wine. You may not want as much as the usual recommendation of six to eight glasses a day, but do give your thirst the frequent opportunity of being quenched with its natural need for simple water.

Wine and Beer
Alcoholic beverages are a part of the ancient metabolic foods. Wine is included in the diet for those who want it. It should only accompany food, however and not be used alone. Otherwise it will go straight to your head. Wine especially is good with foods of all kinds and can help make fruits and vegetables a treat. Modern beers do not seem to be as good as wine for weight reduction but they too can accompany foods. Beers resembling ancient ales may be best. Moderation is the key.

Weigh Yourself
Weigh yourself every morning before eating or drinking anything. As the pounds begin to drop, you will look forward to weighing yourself. And you won't be able to kid yourself that yesterday's weakness (or perceived necessity) for fast fat burgers and shakes didn't matter. Weigh without clothes or the same type clothes, so the clothes weigh close to the same each day.

Daily Journal

Keep a journal of your weigh-ins and daily activities as well as your calories. A notebook or sheets of paper and pen or pencil will do. You can also make a computer spreadsheet. However, the pen or paper is more intimate, portable, and doesn't have to be turned on. Just you and your thoughts are the only energy needed. The spreadsheet is a good idea for charting your calorie energy factor however (see *Maximum Calories*, Chapter 8).

Biosphere

Have houseplants in your home and fresh flowers on the table when you can. Even if you see nothing but urban concrete out your window, you can be in touch with these small offerings of nature. Outside, pause and appreciate your living, breathing environment with sunshine, rain, air, people, plants. Visit the garden center at the supermarket on your way to shop for groceries. This allows your biological body to recall living plants and nature rather than being lost in plastic and cardboard. In the park or your yard, take off your shoes and walk in the grass in your bare feet so you can touch and feel the earth.

Seasons

If you are beginning the diet in the winter, the variety of fruits and vegetables can be limited, especially in smaller towns that may not stock the variety available in metropolitan centers. Never mind, there are still plenty of choices in oranges, apples, pears, tropical fruits, squash, green leafies, grapes and so on. Explore the frozen food case for berries that are not drenched in sugar syrup. Summertime is only a few months away. During the summer especially, you'll feel like you are in paradise on this diet with the abundance of luscious fresh produce to eat.

The Harvest is In

Have plenty of food around your kitchen and dining area. This does *not* mean refined carbohydrate and refined sugar products like shelf cookies and chips. It means large bowls or basketfuls of potatoes, vegetables, fruits, nuts. Let your body know that you are secure. The harvest is in and it is a good harvest.

Reduce Stress

Stress is a big part of our busy lives in more ways than we are aware. Find ways to consciously relax your body. Refuse to worry too much. Worry by itself doesn't solve anything. If you must worry and are the worrying kind, restrict it to a time limit.

Sleep

You'll notice your morning weight decreases more after a good night's sleep. The body at rest is not eating or drinking and can use energy to metabolize, clean up, and get ready for the next day. A good night's sleep repairs body and dreams. You will sleep well on this diet. You will not dream of food as you do on starvation diets because you are not going hungry. Good sleep also adds to your feelings of energy and tranquility. Your nerves and body are relaxed from all the good minerals and vitamins you are getting.

Bath and Shower

The skin, your largest organ, needs clean pores to breathe and to aid metabolism. Clean skin feels better and makes you feel better too. It attracts positive energies. You feel more attractive and so you are. Men have said there's nothing more sexy than a freshly-bathed woman. Women would say the same of men. Simple cleanliness makes you feel attractive and empowered in general.

Pat Yourself on the Back

Physically. Reach up and pat yourself between the shoulder blades. Notice how good it feels as the body relaxes instantly. If you feel lonely and unloved, as many do, know that you can't always have all the attention and approval on demand that you want from friends and family who are busy with managing their own lives and their own daily stresses, especially in a fast-paced world. Develop your hobbies and interests and you will be your own best friend, one who doesn't need to hide behind excess weight and seek comfort in empty foods.

Exercise

Of course, exercise is great for everything about our bodies and minds. But it is not a crucial part of this diet because of reasons mentioned earlier. For one thing, you need to concentrate on your eating. Exercise alone cannot cure or counteract bad food choices. For another, exercise for an overweight body out of shape can cause injury, suffering, and be used as a rationale for not correcting the diet. As you lose weight, you will naturally begin to think about and feel like moving more. Exercise can feel especially good and invigorating after losing excessive fat. Stretching and walking are the best and safest beginning exercises. Exercise should also be enriching to the spirit. Mopping the floor, washing the windows, and mowing the lawn may be good exercise but it is likely not as rewarding to the spirit as a walk in fresh air and sunshine, feeling the world around you, playing a sport you love, taking a new dance class, doing yoga, or working out to your favorite music. Like the diet, exercise should feel good and renew the spirit.

Say No to Fast Fat Foods

These are the fast foods at food chains and packaged convenience foods such as snacks and potato chips. Look at the sample of the Fast Fat Food Menu next. Eating this or a similar menu every day would result a weight of around 300 pounds while the person may feel he or she was not eating all that much. The difference in this menu is the high flour, sugar, and fat content totaling nearly 4,000 calories! Decreasing this menu to 1800 calories to support a weight of around 150 pounds requires dropping 2100 calories worth of food. The whole menu has few vegetables and no fruit no matter how much food you take away. And not listed are hidden additives, preservatives, chemicals, and salt. This is not nutritious or metabolizer efficient and illustrates how just eating less of this kind of food in lower calorie intake really does not work for weight reduction. Hunger will increase as willpower fades. The solution is to replace the fattening food with nutritious food.

The menu also shows that weight reduction requires a multifaceted enlightened approach. The protein amounts are high and the carbohydrate amount is barely within the RDA. Fat and salt are high. Most importantly, the totals are at the expense of excessive calories and mystery ingredients.

Fast Fat Food Menu

C = cup t = teaspoon tr = trace dbl = double patty sl = slice						
med = medium oz = ounce lbs = pounds						
Food	Amt.	Calories	Protein	Carbs	Fat	Choles terol
			grams	grams	grams	milli grams
Breakfast						
Toast	1 sl	65	2	12	1	tr
Butter	1 t	35	tr	tr	4	11
Jam	1 t	20	tr	4	tr	0
Coffee	1 C	5	tr	1	tr	2
Midmorning						
Donut, raised	1	242	4	27	14	4
Coffee	1 C	5	tr	1	tr	2
Lunch						
Cheeseburger	dbl	420	21	35	21	60
Single (295)						
French fries	med	460	6	53	25	0
Milkshake	16 oz	420	11	68	10	37
Before Dinner						
Beer - 2	12 oz	290	2	26	0	0
Potato Chips	6 oz	910	6	60	30	0
Dinner						
Pizza - meat & cheese	3 sl	550	39	62	15	63
3/8 of 12"						
Diet cola	12 oz	4	tr	tr	0	0
Snack						
Ice Cream - vanilla	1 C	270	4	32	7	55
		Calories	Protein	Carbs	Fat	Choles
Total		**3696**	**95**	**381**	**127**	**234**
Weight Rate: Calories /12 = 308 lbs						
RDAs - Recommended Daily Allowances (Average Healthy Amounts)						
		2000-2800	45-65 grams	300-390 grams	50-90 grams	300 milligrm

10 MENU MODELS & FOOD LISTS

Contents

Menu Terms & Explanations

Menus – Days 1-7

Food Substitutions for Menus

Foods to Eat

Foods Not to Eat – LTN Foods

Menu Terms & Explanations

SSSA	Stop Starch & Sugar Addiction The first 3 days of the diet replaces processed manufactured starch and sugar and all flour and refined sugar with fruit sugars, milk sugars, and generous natural carbs.
LTN	Little To No, Little To None, Foods
Level 1 Hunger	The beginning twinges of hunger
Anytime Beverages	Water Coffee Flavorings: No artificial creamers. Use natural cream, half & half, lowfat milk, or powdered milk. Sweeten with raw sugar, demerara sugar, or honey. Tea Flavor with milk, raw sugar, demerara sugar. honey, lemon, if needed. Diet Sugar Free Soda (exception: children should have instead lowfat milk, all-natural fruit juice, water, or naturally flavored water) Cranberry Water 1 C water with 2 T – ¼ C all natural, concentrated cranberry juice Lemon Water 1 C water with 1-2 t lemon juice
Diet Yogurt	Avoid yogurt with added sugar (180-250 calories per 8 oz). Nonfat & lowfat may still have lots of sugar added. Read labels. Diet yogurt to use is lowfat, artificially sweetened and flavored (100-120 calories per 8 oz) Read labels.
All Natural Yogurt, Lowfat	Natural yogurt containing live bacteria and no added sugar beyond milk sugars.
LYD Yogurt	Love Your Diet Yogurt: Mix 2T to ¼C lowfat, flavored, diet yogurt (above) with 8 oz all natural yogurt, above. (Note: Organic does not necessarily mean no added sugar. Read labels.)

Abbreviations

C	Cup or 8 oz measure
oz	ounce
T	Tablespoon
t	teaspoon
lb	pound

MENUS DAYS 1-7
Menu 1
SSSA – Stop Starch & Sugar Addiction

Breakfast
3 eggs, scrambled or boiled with 1 T butter or canola oil and a sprinkle of
paprika
(for lower cholesterol: 1 whole egg plus 3 whites)

Level 1 Hunger Snacks - Morning
1 - 2 C Diet or LYD Yogurt
1 - 2 C fresh sweet cherries – as much as wanted

Lunch
2 - 3 pieces deli chicken, battered, fried or broasted
4 - 8 oz potato wedges or jojos
green salad
OR continue Hunger Snacks

Level 1 Hunger Snacks - Afternoon
1 - 2 C Diet or LYD Yogurt
1 - 2 C fresh strawberries – as much as wanted

Before Dinner Appetizers
Vegetables, fresh, raw: sliced cucumbers, radishes, tomatoes – as much as
wanted

Dinner
4 - 6 oz wild salmon fillet cooked in skillet with olive oil, garlic, lemon
1 C rice with tamari soy sauce
1 - 2 C steamed broccoli and carrots with 1 T lowfat sour cream

Dessert
1 C fresh, raw, sliced strawberries
2 T nonfat whipped topping
2 T chocolate sauce

After Dinner Hunger Snacks
Repeat dessert or see Snacks & Nibblers in *Foods to Eat*

Menu 2
SSSA – Stop Starch & Sugar Addiction

Breakfast
1 - 1 ½ C lowfat cottage cheese
2 or more fresh, raw apricots

Level 1 Hunger Snacks - Morning
1 - 2 C Diet or LYD Yogurt
1 - 2 C fresh, raw, red or black seeded grapes – as much as wanted

Lunch
3 oz tuna with green salad and lowfat dressing
Vegetables, fruit, raw, fresh - baby carrots, apple
OR continue Hunger Snacks

Level 1 Hunger Snacks - Afternoon
1 - 2 C Diet or LYD Yogurt
1 - 2 C fresh, raw, red or black seeded grapes – as much as wanted

Before Dinner Appetizers
Vegetables, fresh, raw: sliced avocado, tomato – as much as wanted

Dinner
1 - 2 chicken leg quarters, fried in olive oil, garlic, fresh rosemary
10 oz baked potato (microwaved) with 2 T lowfat sour cream and chopped green onion
1 - 2 C steamed asparagus with 1 T lowfat sour cream

Dessert
Banana Split: 1 banana
½ C no sugar added vanilla or chocolate ice cream
2 T chocolate sauce
2 T peanuts

After Dinner Hunger Snacks
Repeat dessert or see Snacks & Nibblers in *Foods to Eat*

Menu 3
SSSA – Stop Starch & Sugar Addiction

Breakfast
3 eggs, scrambled or boiled with 1 T butter or canola oil and a
sprinkle of paprika
(for lower cholesterol: 1 whole egg plus 3 whites)

Level 1 Hunger Snacks - Morning
1 - 2 C Diet or LYD Yogurt
1 - 3 raw, fresh sweet dark plums

Lunch
1 C cottage cheese
Vegetables, raw, fresh – sliced cucumber, sweet red pepper – as much as
wanted
OR continue Hunger Snacks

Level 1 Hunger Snacks - Afternoon
1 - 2 C Diet or LYD Yogurt
1 - 3 dried dates or figs

Before Dinner Appetizers
Fruit, vegetables, fresh, raw: sliced sweet red pepper, cucumber, black olives
As much as wanted

Dinner
4 - 6 oz fish fillet cooked in olive oil with garlic & lemon
10 oz baked sweet potato, microwaved, with 1 T butter or margarine
1 C steamed Brussels sprouts with 1 T lowfat sour cream

Dessert
1 C instant no sugar, artificially sweetened chocolate pudding
2 T nonfat whipped topping

After Dinner Hunger Snacks
See Snacks & Nibblers in *Foods to Eat*

Daily Menu 4

For changes in menus, see *Food Substitutions* and *Foods to Eat*. You can also repeat favorite menus or menu items. However, keep selections balanced in nutrition with high protein and lots of fruits and vegetables daily.

Breakfast
½ C dry measure oatmeal. Cover w/water and microwave 2 minutes
Add 1 t raw sugar, 2 T chopped apple, ½ C lowfat milk
1 egg boiled served with 1 t butter or margarine and sprinkled with paprika

Level 1 Hunger Snacks - Morning
Peanuts, raisins, grapes. See also *Snacks & Nibblers* in *Foods to Eat*

Lunch
1 C LYD yogurt and ½ C fresh blueberries
Green salad w/lowcal dressing – as much as wanted

Level 1 Hunger Snacks - Afternoon
Same as morning

Before Dinner Appetizers
Vegetables, fresh, raw: sweet peppers, olives, avocado, tomato
as much as wanted

Dinner
2 - 3 chicken thighs, fried in olive oil & garlic, with rosemary
10 oz baked potato with 2 T lowfat sour cream
1 - 2 C fresh broccoli, steamed, 1 T sour cream

Dessert
Apple Delight: 1 apple, sliced. Add 1 t demerara sugar & cinnamon
Microwave 30 sec.
Serve with 1/2 C no sugar added vanilla ice cream or cream

After Dinner Hunger Snack Repeat Dessert

Daily Menu 5

For changes in menus, see *Food Substitutions* and *Foods to Eat*. You can also repeat favorite menus or menu items. However, keep selections balanced in nutrition with high protein and lots of fruits and vegetables daily.

Breakfast
1 C lowfat cottage cheese
1 slice whole wheat toast, bakery fresh, no preservatives (See *Love Your Diet Recipes* for best bread)

Level 1 Hunger Snacks - Morning
Sunflower seeds and raisins. See also *Foods to Eat: Snacks & Nibblers*

Lunch
1 - 2 C LYD Yogurt
Vegetables, raw sliced, cucumbers, tomatoes, as much as wanted

Level 1 Hunger Snacks - Afternoon
Same as morning

Before Dinner Appetizers
Vegetables, fresh, raw, sweet peppers, tomato
4 oz dry red table wine – cabernet sauvignon

Dinner
1 slice bakery fresh French bread with olive oil, butter, garlic
6 oz T-bone steak, cooked in olive oil, garlic, with mushrooms
10 oz baked potato with 2 T sour cream
1 C steamed zucchini and spinach leaves with 1 T sour cream
4 oz cabernet sauvignon

Dessert
Peaches and Cream: 1 - 2 raw fresh sliced peaches, 1 t raw honey, 2 T cream

After Dinner Hunger Snack Repeat Dessert

Daily Menu 6

For changes in menus, see *Food Substitutions* and *Foods to Eat*. You can also repeat favorite menus or menu items. However, keep selections balanced in nutrition with high protein and lots of fruits and vegetables daily.

Breakfast
1 C lowfat cottage cheese
1 slice whole wheat toast, bakery fresh, no preservatives

Level 1 Hunger Snacks - Morning
1 C LYD Yogurt
1 C fresh sweet cherries – as much as wanted

Lunch
1 - 3 oz tuna on green salad
OR Continue Hunger Snacks

Level 1 Hunger Snacks - Afternoon
1 - 2 C LYD Yogurt

Before Dinner Appetizers
Fruit, fresh, red or black grapes with seeds – as much as wanted
4 oz Italian Chianti wine

Dinner
1 - 2 C spaghetti in mushroom sauce, homemade
Parmesan cheese topping
2 slices bakery fresh French bread with butter, olive oil, garlic
Green salad with Italian dressing
4 oz Italian Chianti wine

Dessert
1 C gelatin with artificial sugar
1 T whipped topping

After Dinner Hunger Snack
Repeat dessert

Daily Menu 7

For changes in menus, see *Food Substitutions* and *Foods to Eat*. You can also repeat favorite menus or menu items. However, keep selections balanced in nutrition with high protein and lots of fruits and vegetables daily.

Breakfast

3 - 4 whole wheat pancakes, homemade, with diced apple.
with natural maple syrup

Level 1 Hunger Snacks - Morning

Apple or orange

Lunch

1 C lowfat cottage cheese
Green salad or sliced raw vegetables – as much as wanted

Level 1 Hunger Snacks - Afternoon

1 - 2 C LYD Yogurt

Before Dinner Appetizers

Vegetables, fresh, raw, sliced cucumber and sweet pepper – as much as wanted

Dinner

1 Cornish game hen stuffed with rice
1 C rice with tamari soy sauce
1 C steamed cabbage wedges and carrots with 1 T sour cream

Dessert

1 slice no sugar apple pie
½ C no sugar added ice cream

After Dinner Hunger Snack

Repeat dessert

Food Substitutions for Menus
Food Substitutions
& Protein Amounts
Anytime Beverages listed in *Menu Terms and Definitions* at beginning of chapter.
See also *Foods to Eat.*

Breakfast - Choose food equal to 15-20 grams (gr) protein

1 large egg – 6 gr protein	1 C cottage cheese – 28-30 gr protein	Fruits, raw, fresh
3 eggs – 18 gr protein	1 C Diet or LYD Yogurt – 8-11 gr protein	Whole wheat toast
1 egg yolk – 2.7 gr protein	1 C High Protein Drink – 12-15 gr	To-cook oatmeal
1 egg white – 3.6 gr protein	4 oz meat, poultry, fish -- 25 gr protein	Natural fruit juice
	1 C lowfat milk – 8 gr protein	

Morning Hunger Snacks - Choose food equal to 8-10 grams protein

Protein foods same as breakfast	Fruit – raw, fresh, juicy	Seeds, nuts
	Vegetables – raw, fresh, sliced	Dried fruit

Lunch – Choose food equal to at least 8-10 grams protein

Protein foods same as breakfast	4 oz poultry, meat, seafood – 25 gr protein	Vegetables/salad
Potatoes – wedge or baked	Flatbread, pita	Fruit, raw, fresh
Beans, rice	Tortillas	Hunger snacks

Afternoon Hunger Snacks – Choose food equal to 8-10 grams protein
Same as morning hunger snacks. Eat at Level 1 Hunger.

Before Dinner Appetizers – Curb appetite while preparing dinner

Hummus	Vegetables, raw – sweet peppers,	Fruits, fresh, raw
French bread, bakery fresh	olives, celery, radishes, cucumbers,	melons, peaches,
Whole wheat bread, bakery	tomatoes,	Berries, apple,
	See fruits and vegetables lists in *Calorie Counter*	

Dinner – Choose food equal to 20+ grams protein

Natural "heavy-duty" carbs:	Poultry, seafood, lean meat	Vegetables - cooked

potatoes, rice, beans, yams, sweet potatoes	4 oz – average 25 gr protein French bread, bakery fresh

Desserts – Control (LTN) refined white sugar and manufactured foods

Artificially-sweetened	Fruits, raw, fresh	Natural cream
Ice cream, pies, pudding, gelatin	Raw honey and demerara sugar	Whipped topping
Sometimes – yeast donuts	Chocolate sauce	

After Dinner Snack

Satisfy any hunger with Snacks and Nibblers listed in Foods to Eat or repeat dessert.

Foods to Eat

Protein Foods
Poultry – Chicken, Turkey, Duck
Fish – All Varieties, fresh, frozen
Shellfish – Shrimp, Prawns, Lobster, Oysters,
Scallops, Crab
Meat – Beef, Pork (lean), Wild Game (deer, elk),
Buffalo
Dairy Products
Milk – 1%
Cottage Cheese - 1%
Yogurt – Diet Lowfat, Artificially Sweetened – 100
calories
Yogurt –LYD, Love Your Diet Yogurt – All natural,
no added
sugar yogurt, mixed with 2T – ¼ C Diet Yogurt,
150 calories
Eggs - Fresh, Low Cholesterol
Nutrition Drinks - Flavored, whey, soy protein

Fruit - All Varieties, Fresh, Raw

**Vegetables - All Varieties, Fresh, Raw or
Cooked**

Potatoes (Tubers)
White Potatoes
Sweet Potatoes
Yams

Grains
Rice - Natural, Brown or White, To cook, Non
instant
Cereal - Natural Whole grain, To cook
Oatmeal
Whole Wheat
Mixed Grain

Anytime Beverages
Water
Coffee
Tea
Diet Soda
Milk – Lowfat
Lemon or Cranberry Water

Sometimes Beverages
Wine
Beer

Condiments
Sour Cream
Mustard,
Soy Sauce
Cocktail Sauce
Lemon Juice, fresh
Sauces for Meat
Herbs, Spices
Horseradish

Desserts
Fruit
Puddding, GelatinNonsugar
Whipped Topping
Cream
Ice Cream non-sugar
Honey
Chocolate Sauce

Beans (Legumes), Home cooked, all varieties

Sweeteners
Sugar - Raw, Unrefined
Demerara Sugar, type of raw sugar
Turbinado Sugar, type of raw sugar
Honey
Natural Maple Syrup

Fats, Oils
Olive Oil – Cold press, First press
Butter
Canola Oil & Canola Margarine
Butter & Yogurt Margarine

Snacks & Nibblers
Nuts, Seeds
Fruits, Vegetables
Popcorn, Airpopped
Raisins, Dried Fruit

Supplements
Vitamin Mineral Tablet
Brewer's Yeast
Protein Drink

Sometimes Foods (every 4 to 7 days)
Bakery Bread - Yeast Leavened, French, Italian, Wh.
Wheat
Pasta & Sauce - Homemade Meals
Breads – Unleavened, Pita, Tortillas, Tacos
Pancakes - Whole Wheat w/Fruit & Natural Maple
Syrup
Pizza
Submarine Sandwiches – Bakery Loaf Bread
    homemade or Fast Food Lean, Turkey, Lean
Ham, Vegetables
Batter dipped in Tempura Flour, Fried in Olive Oil,
Shrimp,
    Oysters, Onions, Vegetables

Go Easy Foods

Sweeteners
Cereals
Chocolate Sauce
Chocolate bar
Cream
Ice Cream
Cheese
Breaded, Batter dipped

Wine
Butter
Oils
Fats
Salt
Pasta
Breads

Foods Not to Eat – LTN Foods

What Not to Eat – The LTN (Little to No) Foods

FOOD/INGREDIENT	Type	Average Calories/Amount
Bagels	All varieties.	80/oz
Biscuits	Made with flour, baking powder.	100/oz
Biscuits	Made from refrigerated dough.	90/oz
Breads	Packaged and preserved.	70-80/oz
Breads, Bakery Sometimes Food	OK: Fresh, yeast leavened, no preservatives or additives.	80/oz
Brownies	Regular or lowfat.	100/oz
Cakes	All varieties.	105/oz
Candy & candy bars	All varieties.	Various
Canned foods	Soup, beans, pasta. Exceptions: vegetables & fruit in natural juices.	Various
Carbonated sodas	Sweetened with sugar syrups. High sugar count.	150/12 oz 13 per oz
Cereals	Ready-to-eat. Sugars, additives.	80-120/oz
Chips	Tortilla, nacho, corn, potato.	140-150/oz
Cookies	All varieties.	100/oz
Corn syrup products	Added as sweetener to prepared foods.	Various
Crackers	All varieties - cheese, saltine, graham, wheat, rye.	120-140/oz
English muffins	All varieties.	65/oz
Flour – Sometimes Food	Flour and flour products. Gluten additives for fillers.	Various
Food Additives	Starches - flour, gluten, cornstarch, sugar, corn syrup. Artificial colors and flavorings. Preservatives.	Various
French toast	All varieties.	75/oz
Frozen dinners	All varieties. Artificially flavored. Flour & thickeners. High salt.	25-200/oz
Frozen foods	All varieties. Artificially sweetened and flavored. Flour & thickeners. High salt.	Various

	Exceptions: Fish, batter coated fish, vegetables, fruit, natural, nonsweetened. Whipped topping. Meatless patties. Soy and vegetable burgers.	
Gravies	All varieties.	30-100/1/4 C
Hot dogs & frankfurters	All varieties. Preservatives.	140/each
Ice cream	Fully sweetened with sugars and syrups. High sugar count. Chemical preservatives & flavors. Exceptions: all natural, no sugar added, artificial sweetener OK, regular or lowfat OK.	280/8 oz cup 35 per oz
Juice Drinks	Added water, flavorings, sugar, corn syrup, high sugar count	115/8 oz 14 per oz
Liquors	Gin, vodka, rum, whiskey.	100/1.5 oz
Luncheon meat	Bologna, salami, beef, pork, chicken, turkey. Preservatives.	60-90/oz
Margarines & shortenings	High in trans fats or hydrogenated oils.	75-115/T
Meats, preserved, cured	All varieties. Luncheon meat, sausage, ham, hot dogs, bacon.	100/oz
Milk shakes	Fully sweetened with sugars and syrups. Artificial flavors.	350/10 oz 35 per oz
Muffins	All varieties.	80-85/oz
Packaged foods & dinners Dry, canned, frozen	TV dinners. Canned, frozen macaroni, rice, spaghetti, pudding. Additives. Exception: Artificially sweetened puddings and gelatin desserts for dieting.	Various
Pancakes/waffles – Sometimes Food	All varieties. Exception: homemade once a week.	40-80/oz
Pasta – Sometimes Food	All varieties. Exception: OK every 4 -7 days.	25/oz
Pastries	All varieties-doughnuts, Danish, éclairs, cinnamon rolls, toaster pastries.	105-120/oz
Pies	All varieties. Exception: No sugar added fruit OK once a week.	75/oz

Potato chips	All varieties.	150/oz
Pretzels	All varieties.	110/oz
Rolls	Hot Dog, hamburger, dinner.	80/oz
Sausages.	Salami, pork, beef, dry.	120/oz
Snack cakes	Packaged, crème-filled	105/oz
Soup	All prepared varieties. Additives. High salt.	100-200/oz
Spaghetti – Sometimes Food	All varieties. Exception: OK every 4-7 days, homemade.	25/oz
Syrup	Corn syrup. Imitation maple and artificial flavorings.	60/T
Tacos, Tortillas, Pita – Sometimes	OK every 4-7 days.	Various
Yogurts	High sugar & calories	230/8 oz

Reference Sources

Ancient Mesopotamian Foods. Ancient Egypt.
    http: www.foodtimeline.org/foodfaq3.html
Baines, Dr. John. *Ancient Egypt Timeline.*
    http:www.bbc.co.uk/history/ancient/egyptians/timeline.shtml
Billard, Jules B., Editor. *Ancient Egypt. Discovering its Splendors.*
    Washington, D.C.: National Geographic, 1978
Gebhart, Susan E. and Robin G. Thomas. *Nutritive Value of Foods.*
    Rev. Ed. Oct. 2002. Home and Garden Bulletin Number 72. U.S.
    Department of Agriculture. Agricultural Research Service.
    Washington, D.C.: GPO, 2002.
Hunter, Erica C.D. *First Civilizations*, Rev. Ed. New York: Facts on File,
    Inc. Oxfordshire, UK: Andromeda Oxford, Ltd., 2003.
Kirschmann, Gayla J., Nutrition Search, Inc., John D. Kirschmann,
    Director.*Nutrition Almanac.* 4th Edition. New York: McGraw-Hill,
    1996.
U.S. Department of Agriculture, Agricultural Research Service. 2005.
    *USDA National Nutrient Database for Standard Reference,
    Release 18, 20.*
Nutrient Data Laboratory:
    http://www.nal.usda.gov/fnic/foodcomp/search/
Wells, Spencer. *The Journey of Man: A Genetic Odyssey*. Princeton,
    N.J.: Princeton University Press, 2002.

ABOUT THE AUTHOR

K.J.R. Alexander is a teacher, researcher, and writer who lives with her family in Oregon. She is the author of the *Love Your Diet* series of books.

www.ingramcontent.com/pod-product-compliance
Lightning Source LLC
Chambersburg PA
CBHW071219280526
45787CB00002B/726